Learning IOM/HMD

Learning
IOM/HMD

Implications of the Institute of Medicine
and Health & Medicine Division
Reports for Nursing Education

Fourth Edition

Anita Finkelman, MSN, RN

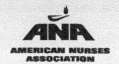

American Nurses Association
Silver Spring, Maryland

2017

American Nurses Association
8515 Georgia Avenue, Suite 400
Silver Spring, MD 20910-3492
1-800-274-4ANA
http://www.NursingWorld.org

The America Nurses Association (ANA) is the premier organization representing the interests of the nation's 3.6 million registered nurses. ANA advances the nursing profession by fostering high standards of nursing practice, promoting a safe and ethical work environment, bolstering the health and wellness of nurses, and advocating on health care issues that affect nurses and the public. ANA is at the forefront of improving the quality of health care for all.

The opinions in this book reflect those of the authors and do not necessarily reflect positions or policies of the American Nurses Association (ANA).

Library of Congress Cataloging-in-Publication Data available on request.

978-1-55810-683-3	print	SAN: 851-3481	07/2017
978-1-55810-684-0	ePDF		
978-1-55810-685-7	EPUB		
978-1-55810-686-4	Kindle		

First printing: July 2017.

Brief Contents

Contents

Part I: The IOM/HMD Reports and Nursing Education

Part II: Incorporating the Core Competencies into Nursing Education

About the Author

Anita Ward Finkelman, MSN, RN, a nurse educator and consultant, is Visiting Lecturer, Nursing Department, Recanati School for Community Health Professions Faculty of the Health Sciences, Ben-Gurion University of the Negev, Beersheba, Israel. She has held several faculty positions; most currently she was visiting faculty at Northeastern University, Bouvé College of Health Sciences and School of Nursing, where she taught and also served as faculty chair for AACN accreditation renewal for BSN and Master's Programs and new accreditation for DNP Program. Prior to this position, she was an Assistant Professor of Nursing at the University of Oklahoma College of Nursing and served as Director of Undergraduate Curriculum and Associate Professor of Clinical Nursing at the University of Cincinnati College of Nursing. Her BSN is from Texas Christian University, master's degree in psychiatric–mental health nursing, clinical nurse specialist from Yale University, and post-master's graduate work in health care policy and administration from George Washington University. Additional work in the area of health policy was completed as a fellow of the Health Policy Institute, George Mason University.

Ms. Finkelman's more than thirty-five years of nursing experience include clinical, educational, and administrative positions, and considerable experience developing online courses and curriculum. She has authored many books and journal articles, served on editorial boards, and lectured on administration, quality improvement, health policy, education, and psychiatric–mental health nursing, both nationally and internationally, particularly in Israel for the Hebrew University Hadassah School of Nursing; Haifa University, where she served on the interprofessional advisory committee for the first Evidence-Based Practice Center in Israel; and Ben Gurion University in Beersheba, Israel, where she developed a collaborative health care profession study-abroad program with Northeastern University.

She is also a consultant to publishers and health care organizations in the areas of distance education and development of Internet products. Recent textbook publications include *Professional Nursing Concepts: Competencies for Quality Leadership* (fourth edition to be published in 2017, Jones & Bartlett Learning), *Quality Improvement: A Guide for Integration in Nursing* (2018, Jones & Bartlett Learning), *Leadership and Management for Nurses: Core Competencies for Quality Care* (2016, Pearson Education, Inc., 3rd ed.), *Case Management for Nurses* (2011, Pearson Education, Inc.), and a number of other books, chapters, and journal articles on leadership and management, health policy, education, international health care, community health, and psychiatric–mental health nursing.

Preface

This second edition of *Learning IOM/HMD: Implications of the Institute of Medicine and Health & Medicine Division Reports for Nursing Education* continues the dialogue about the *Quality Chasm* reports begun with the first edition in 2007. There have been many opportunities through presentations at conferences and workshops across the United States and abroad to talk with many nurse educators, staff development professionals, and clinicians from health care organizations about the implications of these critical reports and nursing education. This led to expansion of this book.

Throughout this book, as well as in the *Quality Chasm* reports, there is an important factor: *This cannot be done alone.* Nursing needs more dialogue and more collaboration—partnerships among nurses, particularly between nurse educators and nurses in practice, and partnerships with our colleagues in other health care professions. Students and patients require this. We are a practice profession, and this is where our emphasis should be.

How does this edition compare to the first? Publishing two volumes, one for nurse educators (*Teaching IOM-HMD*) and this one for students, continues. This is due to continued interest from educators who have requested a student version.

Retaining the same format and structure, this edition updates and expands content. More reports that are relevant to nursing have been included. There are updates to and expansion of content on health care reform and its implications for quality improvement, as well as connection of the reports to nursing standards and ethics. There is more discussion of the five health care core competencies, continued recognition of

Quality and Safety Education for Nurses (QSEN), and more examples of teaching-learning strategies. While these strategies are more explicitly emphasized and interwoven into this book, they have also informed both titles. These strategies are aligned with the Carnegie Foundation's 2010 report *Educating Nurses: A Call for Radical Transformation*, which promotes student engagement and movement away from lecture-driven education.

There is continued recognition of the importance of *Quality Chasm* reports for health care delivery and their ongoing implications for nursing. There is great need for nursing to make changes in nursing education to better serve our students and consequently their employers—but more importantly, to provide quality care for all patients who require it and support health in our communities. In addition, the content has relevance for staff educators who must assure that their staff is competent in the five health care profession core competencies.

Overview of This Edition

As described previously, the fourth edition consists of two volumes. *Teaching IOM/HMD*, is primarily for faculty in nursing education programs and staff educators in practice settings.

The revised edition of *Learning IOM/HMD* is a shorter version of *Teaching IOM/HMD* and is primarily for students, either undergraduate or graduate.

- **Part I** covers background information needed to better understand the many changes in health care delivery and their impacts on the nursing profession and nursing education, and provide guidance for faculty in preparing learning experiences for students. The chapters focus on the following:
    - **Chapter 1** sets the context for the book with an overview of the critical *Quality Chasm* series of reports and other reports issued by the IOM and the HMD.
    - **Chapter 2** discusses health care reform and its connection to the quality improvement initiative.
    - **Chapter 3** provides information about the relationship of the *Quality Chasm* reports, nursing standards and ethics, and other significant nursing policy statements.

- **Part II** is the longest and most detailed part of each book and discusses content and teaching-learning strategies for each of the five health care professions core competencies:

Acknowledgments

I would like to thank my family: Fred, Shoshannah, and Deborah Finkelman. Thank you to previous coauthor Carole Kenner for the first through third editions. Thanks to Elizabeth Karle for assistance with administrative matters for several of the editions. Finally, special thanks to Joe Vallina and Eric Wurzbacher of ANA's book publishing program for all their help in supporting this initiative and preparing the manuscripts for publication. Patients and students have also helped guide the development of this discussion to improve patient care and our teaching.

Part I

The IOM/HMD Reports and Nursing Education

Summaries, Recommendations, and Implications

In 1970, the Institute of Medicine (IOM), a nonprofit organization based in Washington, DC, was established. In 2015, the IOM underwent a name change to become the Health and Medicine Division (HMD) of the National Academies of Sciences, Engineering, and Medicine (collectively "the Academies"). In this book, references to the IOM prior to June 2015 will remain IOM, and after this date references and content related to this organization will be referred to as HMD (HMD 2016a). The HMD acts as an advisor to the nation to improve health by providing evidence-based advice to policymakers, professionals, educators, and the public, as did the IOM. It cannot make laws or regulations; rather, it makes recommendations. When asked to examine problems, it invites a panel of experts to address specific questions related to the problem and then publishes the panel's final report of its findings and recommendations. Many of them are critically important to nursing practice and education.

As noted in the preface, part I sets the context for the teaching-learning strategies of part II. Of primary importance are discussions of a selection of the many reports issued by the IOM and the HMD that are most relevant to nursing. Part I also provides the background information needed to better understand the many changes in the health care arena and their impacts on quality improvement, the nursing profession, and nursing education, and provides guidance for faculty in preparing learning experiences for their students:

- Chapter 1 sets the context for the book with an overview of sixty-eight IOM and HMD nursing-relevant reports. These start with the critical *Quality Chasm* series of reports that began in 1999 and continued through the game-changing 2010 report, *The Future of Nursing*, and several others until 2016. To facilitate reference to these discussions, they are arranged chronologically and grouped into nine categories: quality care; diversity, disparity, and health literacy; leadership; public and community health; research and evidence-based care; health care informatics; nursing; best practices; and health care professions education. Concluding the chapter is a discussion of some key implications of these reports for clinical care.

- Chapter 2 discusses health care reform and its connection to the quality improvement initiatives.

- Chapter 3 provides information about the relationship between the *Quality Chasm* reports, nursing standards and ethics, and other significant nursing policy statements.

1

Summaries, Recommendations, and Implications of the Reports for Nursing

In 1997, President Clinton established a short-term commission called the Advisory Commission on Consumer Protection and Quality in the Healthcare Industry. The purpose of this commission was to advise President Clinton about the status of the health care delivery system, changes related to quality, consumer protection, and the availability of necessary services (Wakefield 1997). The commission investigated many aspects of quality care and the changes needed to improve care, and published a report, *Quality First: Better Health Care for All Americans*, of its findings (Advisory Commission on Consumer Protection and Quality in the Healthcare Industry 1999). The commission had no idea that it was opening a Pandora's box and that its work would lead to a comprehensive examination of US health care, resulting in numerous health care quality reports and recommendations, including the need for change in health care professions education. After this report from the President's Commission, *To Err Is Human* (Kohn, Corrigan, and Donaldson 1999) became the first in the *Quality Chasm* series of reports, and the IOM was asked to further examine health care quality, respond to issues identified in the 1999 Advisory Commission's report, and identify strategies to improve health care quality over the next ten years. This work continues now, more than seventeen years later.

Many of the earlier reports are described in the following sections, as are more current reports that focus on quality care, diversity and disparity, leadership, public and community health, research and evidence-based practice (EBP), health informatics, nursing, best practices for better health, health care education, and many other issues that are highly relevant to nursing education and practice. The work done by this organization is also highly significant for nursing education and practice, as demonstrated by the following information about some of its landmark reports on the quality of care and subsequent discussion of the implications of those reports. This summary focuses on some of the reports and is divided into focus areas, but it does not represent all of the reports. The past and current reports may be accessed through the HMD website, viewed online or downloaded as PDFs (http://www.nationalacademies.org/hmd/Reports.aspx).

Why should nurse educators pay attention to the *Quality Chasm* series and the work done to develop them? The 1983 report *Nursing and Nursing Education: Public Policy and Private Actions* recommended that nursing research be included in mainstream health research (IOM 1983). This recommendation led to the creation of the National Center for Nursing Research (NCNR) within the National Institutes of Health (NIH) in 1993, which later became the National Institute of Nursing Research (NINR). This is an example of a major impact on nursing. The NINR celebrated its thirtieth anniversary in 2016 and published a new strategic plan, *Advancing Science, Improving Lives: A Vision for Nursing Science*, identifying four focus areas for nursing research (NINR 2016):

1. **Symptom science.** Promoting personalized health strategies
2. **Wellness.** Promoting health and preventing illness
3. **Self-management.** Improving quality of life for individuals with chronic conditions
4. **End-of-life and palliative care.** The science of compassion

In 2016, NINR director Patricia Grady commented,

> *as we look toward the future of nursing science, NINR will continue to evolve in supporting scientific research, facing new health challenges and needs as they emerge. Emerging needs and opportunities go hand-in-hand—thus, NINR's goals are to identify proactive, innovative solutions to these challenges, which will allow NINR to continue to advance cutting-edge science to improve the health of the Nation. However, NINR is aware we cannot predict precisely where science, innovation, or health challenges will take us. Therefore, it is important to remember that this strategic plan is a flexible, living document. NINR will regularly assess the emerging body of science and health challenges that arise, and adapt the Institute's research strategies to meet these needs.* (Grady 2016)

Nursing education is very involved in nursing research, from offering content and experiences related to research and EBP for all students, to guiding student research and supporting and guiding faculty research. Nursing research in health care organizations (HCOs) has increased since the establishment of NINR.

The HMD report recommendations make a difference in health care policy and practice, funding, and education. These reports are at the center of the current restructuring of health care systems, particularly in relationship to quality improvement (QI) and the movement toward interprofessional team collaboration. They influence funding from public and private sources, education, and health policy agencies and professional organizations. Their content and recommendations should be integrated as appropriate in all nursing education programs.

The reports must also be viewed within the nursing context. How the reports are viewed by nurses and whether they are implemented by the nursing profession is influenced by the current status of nursing practice and education, which may impede integration of critical, current views of health care and the need for change and improvement. Why is this so? There has long been a wall between nursing education and nursing practice. We (not just nurses but all health care professionals) need to take a serious look at changes, even if we are satisfied with the status quo. The reports and their recommendations indicate that health care professionals need to combine education and practice in order to improve care. The reports on quality also provide a platform for improvement in health care, which should be reflected in efforts to improve collaboration between education and practice. This book is predicated on change and acceptance of the need to move forward and work more collaboratively with our colleagues from all health care professions in all health care settings.

Quality Care

Since 1999, IOM/HMD has published many major reports that focus primarily on general aspects of quality care. This was the initial focus of the health care reports. The reports are significant as they turned the nation's attention to the status of health care quality and the need for improvement. The following summaries highlight the major, initial reports in the *Quality Chasm* series and subsequent reports that built on the quality framework developed in the initial reports.

To Err Is Human (1999)

To Err Is Human describes the national patient safety problem and has significantly influenced the public's view of health care. This report was the result of the request from President Clinton's commission on health. Ensuring patient safety requires a comprehensive approach, and we cannot rely on a single solution. This report is known for its recognition that the United States had a higher rate of health care delivery errors than expected.

Next to recognition of the high level of errors, the most important conclusion from the report is the need to change to a nonpunitive, blame-free health care environment. If a survey were to ask health care providers what they think is the most common type of error, the prevailing response would probably be individual provider errors. Providers would also point out that they are at risk if they report these errors.

This is a simplistic view of errors and avoids addressing the more significant effects of systems and processes on errors. "Building safety into processes of care is a more effective way to reduce errors than blaming individuals" (Kohn, Corrigan, and Donaldson 1999, 4). It is much easier to blame an individual, and this punitive approach has been a tradition in HCOs. It has left us with an environment of fear in which individual staff members are reluctant to report errors or near misses. It ignores the critical fact that errors also provide important information about how the system is working and keeps practitioners from using this information to improve care.

Latent or unnoticed errors are the most problematic errors, and they can later lead to more complex errors. It is, however, much easier to address active errors, which are more visible, and miss the latent errors or errors that are not under the control of the direct care staff, such as equipment problems, environmental issues, and management decisions. Instead, root cause analysis, a standardized method of analyzing errors, should be conducted to determine individual practices and system problems that result in errors. The expectation is that HCOs will then analyze the data and use the analysis to develop interventions that will eliminate or at least reduce the system problems that compromise patient safety. Safe care does not guarantee that the care is higher quality; however, it does increase the likelihood of quality care. It would be easy to say that a strong regulatory and enforcement approach is the strategy for solving this problem, but there are many other strategies to reduce errors that should also be considered. The report also notes that there is a need for a national mandatory error reporting system, which will provide useful information to improve safety.

To Err Is Human concludes by identifying five principles for the design of safe health care systems: (1) provide leadership, (2) respect human limits in process design, (3) promote effective team functioning, (4) anticipate the unexpected, and (5) create a learning environment. One of the recommendations emphasizes the need to continue examining health care quality, as the reported error rate was most likely a low estimate due to the variation in how hospitals defined or tracked errors. This recommendation led to the next report in the *Quality Chasm* series, which expanded the examination beyond a focus on health care safety to a focus on overall health care quality.

Crossing the Quality Chasm (2001)

Following *To Err Is Human*, the next three reports consider a new health system for the twenty-first century. The first of the three, *Crossing the Quality Chasm* (IOM 2001), describes the nation's health care system as requiring fundamental change. At the same time, it recognizes that the system *has* experienced rapid changes, such as new medical science, new technology, and near-immediate availability of information. Nevertheless, the report states that the health care system is fragmented and poorly organized and does not use its resources efficiently, problems that continue today. This report identifies quality as a system property with six important improvement aims: Health care should be safe, timely effective, efficient, equitable, and patient-centered (STEEEP). All health care constituents or stakeholders, including policymakers, purchasers, regulators, health professionals, health care trustees and management, and consumers, must commit to a national agenda emphasizing these six aims for improvement. The goal is to raise the quality of care.

The report describes a vision of health care by identifying ten rules to guide major stakeholders to reach positive outcomes through collaboration. These rules are drawn from the work of Donald Berwick (2008), who also notes the fundamental differences between the new rules and the current system, as discussed in chapter 4. This report recognizes that although health care safety is critical, it is a component of health care quality, and we need to also understand the broader perspective of quality.

Envisioning the National Healthcare Quality Report (2001)

After completing a more in-depth description of the health care problem, the next concern was routine monitoring of health care quality. The challenge was what to do with the information we were gaining about quality care. This report took the process a step further by proposing a system for annual data collection on the quality of the nation's health care system. There was need for a framework to use for monitoring health care quality. *Envisioning the National Healthcare Quality Report* (Hurtado, Swift, and Corrigan 2001, 2) describes the framework for data collection, and that framework was initially used to annually monitor quality of care, though it has been modified since the original version was developed. This quality care analysis is now compiled annually by the Agency for Healthcare Research and Quality (AHRQ), an agency in the US Department of Health and Human Services (HHS).

The National Healthcare Quality Report "should serve as a yardstick or the barometer by which to gauge progress in improving the performance of the health care delivery system in consistently providing high-quality care" (Hurtado, Swift, and Corrigan 2001, 2). The report does not focus on public health, but instead on health care system performance in providing personal health care (health care for the individual), primarily acute care. In addition, the report discusses health care from a broader perspective than the performance of individual providers such as hospitals. The report notes that the proposed national monitoring should not duplicate systems that many individual HCOs use to measure their own performance. The quality report should assist policymakers and also be accessible and relevant to consumers, purchasers, providers, educators, and researchers. The design of the annual quality report builds on the definition of quality used in the various *Quality Chasm* reports. *Quality* is "the degree to which health services for individuals and populations increase the likelihood of desired health outcomes and are consistent with current professional knowledge" (Lohr 1990, 21).

The quality report follows the most common approach to quality care assessment, derived from Donabedian's (1996) three elements of quality:

structure, process, and outcomes. It is clear that quality health care does not necessarily mean that desired outcomes will always be reached; a patient who receives care below the quality standard may still reach the desired outcomes. In addition, the approach selected for the report recognizes the influence of the patient's desired outcome and preferences on treatment and health care consumerism.

The first annual report was published online in 2003 by the AHRQ. The annual report is a rich source of data, with current updates that can be used to create course content, learning activities, and student examinations of data. The reports are relevant to health policy and should be reviewed by HCOs. The current annual report can be accessed at the AHRQ site (https://www.ahrq.gov/research/findings/nhqrdr/nhqdr15/index.html). As noted later in this part, the annual report on quality now is combined with disparities monitoring, referred to as the QDR (National Quality and Disparities Report). Typically, the health care quality report is published to two years behind the current date due to the time required to collect and analyze data.

Priority Areas for National Action: Transforming Health Care Quality (2003)

Priority Areas for National Action (Adams and Corrigan 2003) adds another building block to the national initiative to improve health care quality. This report recognizes that every aspect of care cannot be assessed annually, and that attempting to do so would not offer any advantage. The increase in chronic conditions in the United States has had a major impact on the health care system and is an important consideration when identifying priority areas. More people are living longer and with chronic illnesses, mostly because of advances in medical science and technology. Many of these patients also have comorbid conditions that increase the complexity of their problems and require more collaborative health care. Three criteria were used to select the priority areas:

1. Impact or extent of burden
2. Improvability or extent of the gap between current practice and evidence-based practice
3. Inclusiveness or relevance of an area to a broad range of individuals

The report initially specified nineteen priority areas. Over time, the priority areas have changed as new needs arise and outcomes in priority areas improve. The current QDR provides details about the current priority areas (AHRQ 2015).

Patient Safety: Achieving a New Standard of Care (2003)

Patient Safety discusses in more detail one recommended strategy for improving patient safety, defined as "freedom from accidental injury" (Aspden et al. 2003, 4). Patient safety improvement requires major changes. Multiple stakeholders must commit to these changes, which include revamping patient information systems. This report continues the examination of safety issues and relates to the recommendations found in *To Err Is Human*. In the process of giving health care, providers need to (1) access complete patient information; (2) understand the implications of environmental factors such as time spent waiting to receive care, bed availability, access to equipment and supplies, space to work, and so on; (3) use information about infectious diseases to decrease patient risk through techniques such as handwashing; and (4) understand the implications of chronic illness. Each of these elements depends on accurate, timely, and accessible information in the form of a comprehensive electronic medical record / electronic health record (EMR/EHR). The EMR/ EHR supports the implementation of best practices and evidence-based care, facilitating standardization of care where appropriate. There is more information on health informatics later in this part and in chapter 8.

Preventing Medication Errors (2006)

The first report in the *Quality Chasm* series, *To Err Is Human*, sounded the alarm for health care providers and for consumers, informing them that there are too many errors in the health care system. *Preventing Medication Errors* focuses on information about several facets involved in medication errors: the drug development system, regulation and distribution issues, relevance of literature on the incidence and costs of medication errors, and prevention strategies (Aspden 2006). Using all this information as background, the report proposes a comprehensive approach to reducing medication errors. This plan requires changes in the health care practice of physicians, nurses, pharmacists, and other health care providers, as well as the Food and Drug Administration (FDA), hospitals and other HCOs, and health-related government agencies.

More current data notes that adverse drug events (ADEs) impact seven hundred thousand emergency department visits and one hundred thousand hospitalizations each year. While in the hospital, 5 percent of patients experience ADEs, making this one of the most common inpatient errors. It is estimated that ambulatory patients may experience more ADEs, but more data are needed to determine how many more (PSNet 2015a). These errors are expensive, with patients requiring additional care, and although not all ADEs are preventable, many are. Chapter 7 includes additional information on ADEs.

The plan for change begins with greater emphasis on the patient-provider relationship—asking patients to assume a more active role in their care, supported by increased education about their medications and more opportunities to ask questions and question medication decisions. As will be noted later, this leads to a greater emphasis on patient-centered care (PCC). Greater standardization of patient medication information is also needed.

The second important component of reforming medication administration is the use of health information technologies (HIT) to prescribe and dispense medications; however, there are risks for errors even when using HIT. The third area of concern is the need to improve medication labeling and packaging. Finally, the plan covers policy issues such as funding for research on medication error prevention and greater efforts by regulatory agencies to guide and enforce standards to reduce medication errors.

Advancing Quality Improvement Research: Challenges and Opportunities (2007) and The State of QI and Implementation Research (2007)

Crossing the Quality Chasm discusses the need for improvement in health care quality. It was followed by *Envisioning the National Healthcare Quality Report*, which describes the framework and process for a national health care quality report. We now have an active annual report that is accessible via the Internet. However, just recognizing that there is a problem in health care quality and collecting annual data on the status of that quality is not sufficient to improve care. *Advancing Quality Improvement Research* (Chao 2007a) and *The State of QI and Implementation Research* (Chao 2007b) explore examples of QI methods, focusing on the non–health care service sector (for example, Six Sigma and Lean Sigma), the integrated health care delivery system (for example, Kaiser Permanente), the hospital perspective, and health care professions' perspectives, such as nursing.

Much remains to be understood about QI and the methods used to analyze improvement. Some of these methods are case reports, systematic reviews, controlled trials, and hybrid quantitative and qualitative reports. This area of research differs from other types in what is considered the "gold standard." Some experts claim that randomized controlled trials (RCTs), considered the gold standard in research methods, do not effectively assess complex social contexts; other experts do not agree. Numerous barriers may obstruct QI and QI research, and we need to gain a better understanding of them. This knowledge could be expanded by both

QI field projects and research that meets acceptable standards of effective QI and research (Chao 2007a).

Transforming Health Care Scheduling and Access: Getting to Now (2015)
This report is a good example of how a national health care need drives the need to examine a problem and arrive at options to improve care. In this situation the driver was a problem with Veteran's Health Administration (VHA) wait times that caused major concern about overall care for veterans (Kaplan, Hamilton Lopez, and McGinnis 2015). The VHA requested that the HMD examine the issue of wait times and access, and this expanded to health care delivery beyond the VHA. The report notes the importance of the identification of the six aims (STEEEP) in *Crossing the Quality Chasm.* Of the six aims, "timely" has received less attention, and yet it is critical to ensuring that patients receive care when they need it. What do we really know about health care access, scheduling, and wait times nationally? The examination and final report focuses on patient-centered care as the critical element in achieving timeliness. It also notes that successful approaches to improvement require a system in which the components are interconnected.

What strategies, policies, and leadership are needed to improve timeliness as one of the STEEEP aims? The report provides innovative examples of how some health care delivery systems have improved timeliness. Some of the report's general themes include issues arising from variations in care practices from state to state and HCO to HCO; concern about delays in treatment and causes; thoughts on standards and how they are applied; the need for research on timeliness in health care delivery; the application of best practices and sharing of best-practice information; and the leadership required to ensure that practice is up to standard and timely.

Diversity, Disparity, and Health Literacy
The following reports focus on the critical concern of equality in health care. In the initial *Quality Chasm* reports it was noted that there might be a problem with disparities in health care. This led to a number of initial reports aimed at achieving greater understanding of diversity in health care. Since the first annual AHRQ report on the status of disparities, which was requested because of the *Quality Chasm* reports, we have learned a great deal and now monitor disparities as well as quality of care in the QDR. We also now include more content on diversity and disparities in our health care profession academic programs and staff education.

Guidance for the National Healthcare Disparities Report (2002)

Guidance for the National Healthcare Disparities Report (IOM 2002) proposed a framework for creating the annual National Healthcare Disparities Report, now published by the AHRQ and available on the Internet (IOM 2002). The *Guidance* report is a companion to the National Healthcare Quality Report. As noted earlier, this report and its analysis are now combined into one report covering quality and disparities, the QDR. It provides a comprehensive national overview of disparities in health care as they affect racial, ethnic, and socioeconomic groups and priority populations. Similar to the National Healthcare Quality Report, the annual disparities report flows from the earlier *Quality Chasm* reports on diversity and disparity in health care.

Unequal Treatment: Confronting Racial and Ethnic Disparities in Health Care (2003)

Unequal Treatment focuses on disparities in health care and their impact on the nation's public health, identifying major concerns about racial, ethnic, geographic, and socioeconomic inequities (Smedley, Stith, and Nelson 2003). Health care disparities occur consistently across a variety of illnesses and delivery services. The findings of the Sullivan Commission (Sullivan 2004), though not one of the HMD reports, are relevant to this topic. The Commission examined disparities in health care and concluded that a key contributor to this growing problem is disparity in the nation's health professional workforce. This imbalance impedes minorities' access to health care and undermines understanding of their needs. The Sullivan Commission suggested that the solution is to increase the number of minorities in health professions. This translates to increased minority admission into professional schools, something the United States has historically failed to accomplish. Many minority students do not have strong basic education prior to entering college, so if they are admitted, they often do not graduate. At-risk students should receive assistance to give them a greater chance of completing the program.

Unequal Treatment indicates that bias, prejudice, and stereotyping can lead to disparities in health care. We need greater education, standardized data collection to further understand the problem, and policies and procedures to eliminate inequities. This was the report that led to the recommendation to monitor disparities. Health care organizations increased staff training on this topic and included it in many curricula, but is this making a difference in practice? Disparities in health care are not caused only by a lack of education about culture, so one should not expect that changes in education alone would make the difference. It is a multifaceted problem and requires multiple strategies—many of which will affect the delivery process.

The problem of disparity in the nursing profession is slowly resolving, but there still are barriers such as funding, faculty diversity, and other concerns related to diversity in students and faculty. Data from the American Association of Colleges of Nursing (AACN) indicate that representation of students from minority backgrounds increased in all types of nursing programs from 2011 to 2015, with the following specific increases during this five-year span: 5 percent in entry-level baccalaureate programs, 6 percent in master's programs, 8 percent in research-focused doctoral programs, and 8 percent in Doctorate of Nursing Practice (DNP) programs (AACN 2016b, 3). The number of men in nursing programs also increased 12 percent during this five-year period. This does not mean that we do not have a diversity problem in the nursing profession, as we still need to increase diversity—but we are headed in the right direction.

Nursing education tends to stress content related to specific cultural groups as the primary method for improving knowledge of disparities, but this may actually lead to more stereotyping and oversimplification of culture (Betancourt et al. 2005). Johnson (2005) comments that you need both the generic and specific approaches. The AACN recognizes the need for more cultural competency resources and provides these resources to assist faculty in developing cultural competency education on its website (http://www.aacn.nche.edu/education-resources/cultural-competency). The National League for Nursing (NLN) also provides diversity resources for health care providers on its website (http://www.nln.org/advocacy-public-policy/issues/diversity). The Health Resources and Services Administration (HRSA) also supports greater understanding of culture and diversity by providing multiple resources on its website (http://www.hrsa.gov/culturalcompetence/index.html).

Health Literacy: A Prescription to End Confusion (2004)

This report notes that in 2004 nearly half of all American adults—90 million people—had difficulty understanding and using health information, and there was a higher rate of hospitalization and use of emergency services among patients with limited health literacy (Nielsen-Bohlman, Panzer, and Kindig 2004). Concern about and emphasis on health literacy has increased since 2004. Limited health literacy may lead to billions of dollars in avoidable health care costs. Health literacy is much more than a measure of reading skills and includes writing, listening, speaking, arithmetic, and conceptual knowledge. Health literacy is defined as "the degree to which individuals have the capacity to obtain, process, and understand basic information and services needed to make appropriate decisions regarding their health" (2). This same definition was included in the Affordable Care Act of 2010 (ACA), indicating that the problem continues today. Even well-educated people with strong reading and writing skills may have trouble understanding a medical form or health care provider instructions regarding a drug or procedure. This is a critical topic for nursing students, both undergraduate and graduate, and for staff education. In identifying health literacy as a new facet of diversity, this report led to a number of other reports that discuss the relevance of health literacy in a variety of health care situations (some of these reports are discussed later in this part). The Centers for Disease Control and Prevention (CDC) provides extensive information on health literacy including a national plan to improve health literacy (http://www.cdc.gov/healthliteracy/index.html). Additional content is also discussed in chapter 4.

Promoting Health Literacy to Encourage Prevention and Wellness: Workshop Summary (2011)

Health literacy has an impact on the use of preventive services. This report emphasizes the need for public and community health professionals to do less just telling people what they should do and emphasizing the value of prevention to individuals and the community. Health literacy plays a critical role in a person's ability to understand important prevention information. Health and well-being are addressed by primary and secondary prevention, but they are also influenced by nonhealth issues such as residence location, work, family, economics, sociocultural factors, and so on. To meet prevention goals people need to be given instructions they can understand, and for some it is helpful to provide methods to measure if they are reaching identified outcomes (Hernandez and Landi 2011). Those who have an illness need information for self-management.

There is another viewpoint of health literacy that is very important today given the US problem with health care disparities. Health literacy is connected to health disparities. When people do not understand health information, they may not receive the care they need or effective care that meets outcomes. Health equity is necessary for effective health literacy, as giving people the same opportunity requires an equal understanding of information. Examples of strategies that have been used to promote health literacy and improve health promotion, which then impact health equity, are discussed in the report.

America's Healthcare Safety Net: Intact but Endangered (2007)

The "safety net" is the part of the health care system that serves many people who have limited resources for care, such as uninsured, vulnerable populations, and Medicaid patients, often patients with very complex medical needs and socioeconomic limitations. Often safety net services are found in academic medical centers, but they may be located in a variety of settings (Ein Lewin and Altman 2007). Since 2007, the US health care system has expanded, and there is more advanced treatment for patients than ever before. Some provide the care because it is mandated by law or stated as part of an organization's mission. In many cases the providers serve a mix of patients: some belong to these vulnerable populations and others do not. *Crossing the Quality Chasm* describes the health care system as fragmented, consisting of a patchwork of service settings such as clinics, physician offices, and multiple HCOs (IOM 2001). The system is also not financially secure. Some safety net hospitals have closed over the last few years, while others are struggling to maintain services and may need to reduce services. Who, then, provides care in the safety net system and for how long? The most common providers are public hospitals, local health departments, community health centers, academic health care centers (not all but most), and specialty services such as AIDS clinics and school health clinics.

The safety net system varies from state to state, and it has managed to survive, although services and quality have been questioned. However, a number of factors may stress these organizations' already weak financial support and have a major impact on care quality, such as the increasing number of uninsured people, inadequate Medicaid funding, and problems with HCOs providing timely and effective care, often due to limited resources. This report discusses policy issues, the health care safety net system, forces affecting the system, and the future viability of the system.

Implications of Health Literacy in Public Health: Workshop Summary (2014)

Health literacy has an impact on the public health essential services: health promotion, health prevention, environmental health, occupational health, disease prevention and screening, disaster preparedness, mobilization, health policy, data collection and dissemination, and workforce training and development. In examining the implications of health literacy on public health, the report makes several key points to support the need for and approaches to increasing health literacy (Hewitt and Hernandez 2014; Rudd 2013). There is a connection between a patient's health literacy skills and health outcomes. There are multiple barriers to access to health information, sometimes including health profession communication (written and oral) and how health care providers engage patients. The health care environment may also present barriers to patient understanding and patient navigation of the health care system. The system needs to do more to improve health literacy, and this needs to be included in health care profession education. Vulnerable populations are at particular risk for health literacy problems. To improve the public sector, the health care system needs to increase workforce awareness and skills, decrease barriers to getting information, improve data collection and sharing, and improve partnerships (Hewitt and Hernandez 2014). The following strategies support health literacy in relation to the public health goals associated with the following ten essential public health services (CDC 2014; Hewitt and Hernandez 2014):

- Monitor health status to identify community health problems.
- Diagnose and investigate health problems and health hazards in the community.
- Inform, educate, and empower people about health problems.
- Mobilize community partnerships to identify and solve health problems.
- Develop policies and plans that support individual and community health efforts.
- Enforce laws and regulations that protect health and ensure safety.
- Link people to needed personal health services and assure the provision of health care when otherwise unavailable.
- Assure a competent public health and personal health care workforce.
- Evaluate the effectiveness, accessibility, and quality of personal and population-based health services.
- Use research to identify new insights and innovation solutions to health problems.

Achieving Health Equity via the Affordable Care Act (2015)

Achieving Health Equity via the Affordable Care Act: Provisions, and Making Reform a Reality for Diverse Patients: Workshop Summary is a source of clear information about the ACA. It focuses on the ACA and the following: Expansion of coverage, delivery systems, and access points; service delivery and payment reform, including the patient-centered medical home model; public-private partnerships; and challenges to the safety net (Anderson and Olson 2015). Due to the complexity of the ACA, it is easy to be distracted from the need for greater equity, which relates to the implementation of the ACA. As is typical in other *Quality Chasm* reports, definitions from previous reports are carried through to current reports; in this case, the definitions of equity and disparities found in *Unequal Treatment*. In addition, the current system is still hospital-focused, although the ACA notes (like many other sources) the need for greater health promotion and prevention for all populations in hospital and otherwise, such as community services. All of the following themes of this report are important to nursing education and practice (5-6):

- The ACA creates many opportunities to reduce health disparities through expanded coverage, reduced costs, improved quality, and other broad-based health care reforms.
- The ACA contains many provisions aimed specifically at reducing health disparities.
- The number of uninsured people in a state can be dramatically reduced, but doing so will require comprehensive and personalized outreach.

Information technologies can be powerful tools to increase insurance coverage and keep people covered, supporting health equity.

The report also covers a few general concepts from the ACA (Anderson and Olson 2015):

- The concept of patient-centered medical home supports health equity.
- Safety net organizations are critical to the reduction of health disparities under the ACA.
- The commitment of a state's elected leaders has a major impact on the state-by-state implementation of the ACA.
- Both bottom-up, community-based efforts and top-down, policy leadership are essential.
- Implementation of the ACA will encounter difficulties, but these difficulties can be expected to decline over time.
- Under the ACA, every part of the health care system has opportunities to promote health equity.
- Achieving health equity is a broader goal than reducing health disparities, but the ACA's focus on health disparities represents a critical step toward equitable coverage and health outcomes for all Americans.

Since the publication of this report, the ACA has experienced multiple problems. Chapter 2 discusses the ACA, its implications, and its uncertain future.

Health Literacy: Past, Present, and Future: Workshop and Summary (2015)
This report provides critical commentary about health literacy and the HHS, health literacy and medications, issues related to health care delivery, and health profession education (Alper 2015a). It also addresses the connection of health literacy issues with technology, population and public health, research, and disparities. This report does not offer recommendations but rather examines the discussions and presentations that focus on the topic in a roundtable discussion with experts, some of which is highlighted in this summary. The gap between what health care providers intend to communicate and what patients and families understand continues. We need to know more about what people need in order to process and understand health information so that we can make appropriate decisions and meet outcomes. It is important to assess what patients understand. All sectors (HCOs, health care professionals, the government, insurers, and so on) need to be engaged in improving health literacy. The HHS has long been interested in health literacy; for example, it established and manages the *Healthy People* initiative. The AHRQ as an agency in the HHS has also invested in efforts to improve health literacy as noted in earlier report summaries in this part. It is clear that national and state health policies must consider the relevance of health literacy. Health literacy is directly related to health care services quality improvement—patients and health care consumers need clear information that they can understand in order to reach the desired health outcomes.

Health literacy is also a critical element of medication use. Without effective literacy the risk of errors is increased. A few areas of concern are directions given to patients, medication labels, and the increased risks when multiple medications are taken. All of these examples are related to self-management, a topic discussed in this book, which is highly relevant to quality care and patient-centered care. More effort is needed to standardize and improve medication labels. There is need for more research about best practices and medication health literacy. Medical jargon is a major problem and barrier. The FDA is an important stakeholder in drug administration, prescription, and over-the-counter (OTC) medication. The National Healthcare Strategy (NQS), discussed in more detail in chapter 2, also includes health literacy improvement.

The ACA would have an impact on vulnerable populations and health literacy by noting the need to improve access to care. Engaging consumers to even enroll in ACA or any successor health care coverage system requires consideration of health literacy. Health care profession education for all major health care professions has increased efforts to improve diversity and disparity learning opportunities, which includes health literacy and its implications for practice and quality care. Another important consideration is the relationship between health literacy and HIT, which is discussed more in other parts of this book

As noted in other reports, population health and public and community health require understanding of the need for effective health literacy and decreased disparities. We need more research on health literacy, but this should not be the most important focus, as we need more information practice and improvement in health literacy. This report also identifies ten attributes of health-literate organizations (Figure 4-2, Alper 2015a, 33.)

Informed Consent and Health Literacy: Workshop Summary (2015)
All fifty states have some legislation related to the requirement of informed consent for treatment (Alper 2015b). Although there is some variation in requirements, they all indicate that if a health care professional or HCO does not follow the state requirements they are liable for negligence or battery, which constitutes medical malpractice. Health care research also has requirements for informed consent. This report reviews the history and critical elements of patient informed consent and also informed consent for research participants. Both emphasize the need for voluntary choice and a clear process for discussing the study with potential participants, with time to ask questions about potential risks and benefits. A standard form should be used that requires the research participant's signature. As noted in many reports on health literacy, the patient or participant needs to fully understand the information, so these forms need to be written in a way that is easily understood. Risk of harm and benefits should be as clear as possible. In general, consent must include clear and timely communication, written and oral, and a clear process that has been reviewed and approved.

Relevance of Health Literacy to Precision
Medicine: Workshop in Brief (2016)
In 2016, the Precision Medicine Initiative was implemented as an initiative that involves multiple government agencies (Alper 2016b). Precision medicine is an approach to health care that includes attention given to individual variability in genes, environment, and lifestyle. The goal is to recruit more than one million volunteer participants to obtain health and genomic data that would be included in a study to better understand precision medicine. This report notes that vulnerable populations such as minorities may gain a lot from the study results, but typically, they are

underrepresented in research and have low health literacy. Genetic literacy is a segment of health literacy and an area that is particularly weak for most Americans. Improving health literacy will help to gain better data for this study, as communicating the need for participants and engaging participants is critical for success.

Health Literacy and Palliative Care (2016)

Palliative care has become more and more important in the health care system with recognition of the need for more holistic care for people with serious illnesses. Limited health literacy has an impact on ensuring quality care for this population that requires complex care management (Alper 2016a). Other important issues in this report are the influences of interpersonal communication, the patient experience, and the need to develop communication skills to support effective health literacy. This also applies to the health care team that needs training to ensure best practice. This report does not make specific recommendations but rather summarizes in-depth discussion and presentations on the topic of health literacy and palliative care.

The Promises and Perils of Digital Strategies in Achieving Health Equity: Workshop Summary (2016)

Use of technology has expanded in health care, and has expanded the consumer's ability to communicate and obtain information about health care. This expansion has the potential to decrease disparities in health care, particularly if the benefits are distributed equitably. The goals of this workshop and its report are to reduce health disparities and promote health equity in the United States using the following methods (Anderson and Olson 2016, 3):

- Using digital health technologies as a population health strategy
- Engaging racial and ethnic minority populations and communities in efforts that use digital health strategies
- Using effective strategies to engage racial and ethnic minority populations and communities in digital health strategies
- Using different types of digital health technologies in these efforts
- Developing digital health strategies

It is important to note that even with all the technology advances people must come first. Community engagement must be an integral part of technology-based interventions that are used to improve health care. Even though the focus here is on health technology and its impact on disparities, there are other important factors that have an impact such as education, transportation, economics, sociocultural environment, and systems.

The Leadership Reports

This section includes only one report that directly addresses leadership, although leadership is related to all the reports; for example, *Keeping Patients Safe: Transforming the Work Environment of Nurses* (Child 2004) discusses transformational leadership, and *The Future of Nursing: Leading Change, Advancing Health* (IOM 2011a) also includes content on leadership. There is greater need for leadership to improve care in all settings.

Leadership By Example: Coordinating Government Roles in Improving Healthcare Quality (2003)

This report explores the characteristics of an infrastructure that will foster quality care (Corrigan, Eden, and Smith 2003). Six government programs—Medicare, Medicaid, State Children's Health Insurance Program (SCHIP), Department of Defense's (DOD) TRICARE and TRICARE for Life programs, the VHA, and Indian Health Services (IHS)—are examined for their quality enhancement processes. These six programs serve about a third of all Americans. The difficulty with implementing the recommendations in the *Quality Chasm* reports across these systems is the lack of reliable, valid indicators of quality in the systems.

This report's analysis stresses the need for the US government to lead in establishing quality performance measures and improving care quality. After this *Quality Chasm* report, much more has been done by the government to lead in QI. The federal government serves in four health care delivery roles, which makes it uniquely suited to move the quality initiative forward.

1. It serves as a *regulator* when it sets minimum acceptable performance standards.

2. It is the largest *purchaser* of care through its six major government health programs, and thus can have a major impact on other purchasers of care.

3. It is a *provider* of care for veterans, military personnel and their dependents, and Native Americans. The federal government can implement model QI programs and gather data about their outcomes—information that could then be used by other providers.

4. It is a *research sponsor*, particularly in applied health services research.

The Public and Community Health Reports

Although most early *Quality Chasm* reports emphasize issues related to acute care, there were several early reports that recognize the importance of the US public health system. Later reports addressed more issues related to public and community health.

The Future of the Public's Health in the 21st Century (2003) and *Who Will Keep the Public Healthy?* (2003)

The Future of the Public's Health in the 21st Century (IOM 2003) and *Who Will Keep the Public Healthy?* (Gebbie, Rosenstock, and Hernandez 2003) focus on public and community health. Reports discussed earlier, *Unequal Treatment* and *Guidance for the National Healthcare Disparities Report*, also relate to public health. These four reports discuss the problems in the public health system and offer recommendations for improvement. Part of the current atmosphere of change is the need to instill a vision of public health, which has been identified as *healthy people in healthy communities* (Guidry et al. 2010). This vision of the future of public health recognizes that "health is a primary good because many aspects of human potential such as employment, social relationships, and political participation are contingent on it" (IOM 2003, 2). Public health affects citizens, their lifestyle, income, work status, mortality and morbidity, education, and family life. But public health has frequently been overlooked in the broad view of the nation's health. *The Future of the Public's Health* discusses the importance of the population health approach, public health systems, infrastructure, partnerships, accountability, evidence, and communication.

Who Will Keep the Public Healthy? (Gebbie, Rosenstock, and Hernandez 2003) addresses public health needs in a world of globalization, rapid travel, scientific and technological advances, and demographic changes, which lead to problems such rapidly spreading infectious diseases (e.g., Ebola virus, Zika virus), disasters, and wars and refugees. Effective response to public health problems requires well-prepared professionals. Public health professionals are prepared to provide care within the community, to collaborate with community members and other partners such as the government, schools, and HCOs to improve population health.

The Association of Schools of Public Health predicts that by 2020 the United States will need 250,000 additional public health workers; as a consequence, there is more interest in public health among all health care professionals (*Orlando Business Journal*, 2008). According to this report, the traditional core components of public health are still important:

epidemiology, biostatistics, environmental health, health services administration, and social and behavioral science.

Leading Health Indicators for Healthy People 2020: Letter Report (2011)
The HHS has requested that the HMD recommend twelve leading health indicators and twenty-four objectives to assist HHS in its determination of leading indicators and objectives for *Healthy People 2020* (IOM 2011c). This report is a good example of how quality reports are connected to other initiatives such as *Healthy People*. The mission of *Healthy People 2020* is to (HHS 2012):

- Identify nationwide health improvement priorities;
- Increase public awareness and understanding of determinants of health, disease, disability, and opportunities for progress;
- Provide measurable objectives and goals applicable at national, state, and local levels;
- Engage multiple sectors to take actions to strengthen policies and improve practices that are driven by the best available evidence and knowledge; and
- Identify critical research evaluation and data collection needs.

The overarching goals for the 2020 version are to:

- Attain high-quality, longer lives free of preventable disease;
- Achieve health equity and eliminate disparities;
- Create social and physical environments that promote good health; and
- Promote quality of life, healthy development, and healthy behaviors across life stages.

Healthy, Resilient, and Sustainable Communities after Disasters: Strategies, Opportunities, and Planning for Recovery (2015)
Disasters often have a major impact on communities, individuals, and populations, both short term and long term. They impact physical, mental, and social well-being. In addition, disasters can be very costly, requiring private and public financial support. This report discusses a strategic framework for building healthy, resilient, and sustainable post-disaster communities and provides operational guidance with strategies to meet the goals of the framework. Disaster recovery requires planning that includes the following elements.

- **Visioning.** Recovery is an opportunity to develop a shared vision of a healthier, resilient, and more sustainable community.
- **Assessment.** Community health assessments and vulnerability assessments should identify important gaps that are then used to identify priorities and strategies.
- **Planning.** Health care individual providers and organizations need to be involved in the planning, with the recognition that potential health impacts recovery decisions.
- **Implementation.** Resources need to be carefully used for full benefit and synergy.

This report provides a visual guide to understanding how to leverage the products of pre-disaster planning processes in order to support a healthy community approach (HMD 2015a, 7).

Communities vary and those with more vulnerable populations have a greater challenge in disaster recovery; for example, preexisting health deficiencies and disparities make it more difficult. State and local government officials need to be involved in planning, and federal officials are also typically included (e.g., HHS, CDC, Federal Emergency Management Administration [FEMA]). There are many community stakeholders who should be involved in planning and response, not only for their input and the services they provide, but also because all levels of training need to be prepared for disaster. Sharing information is critical and planning how this will be done during all stages of a disaster should be established beforehand. A mix of resource needs must be considered, such as financial, health care, workforce, communication processes, transportation, housing, water and food, personal safety, information technology, special care needs for people with chronic diseases, and so on. Planning should also include special needs such as behavioral health and social services. Place-based recovery strategies are required; for example, road and bridge repair, removal of debris, and building new housing, health care facilities, businesses, and schools. Planning and recovery, based on lessons learned also lead to preparing for the next disaster.

The Role and Potential of Communities in Population Health Improvement: Workshop Summary (2015)

It is important to recognize the role of community in improving health. This workshop and its report focus on several strategies directed at this issue (Wizemann and Thompson 2015a). Examples of strategies are youth organizing, community organizing or other types of community participation, and partnerships between the community, organizations, and relevant individuals (educators, health care professionals, and government officials).

This discussion led to the identification of a variety of topics related to community and population health improvement. The ecosystem perspective is important. Storytelling helps us understand problems and solutions and build trust, and communities connect to data better when the data are associated with stories that people can relate to. Breaking down silos and using "we" engages more people in the community. Other issues are discussed such as youth issues, violence, schools and integration, and so on, with a focus on building partnerships. Examples are provided throughout the report.

Spread, Scale, and Sustainability in Population Health: Workshop Summary (2015)

This workshop and its report focus on: the meanings of the spread and scale of programs, policies, practices, and ideas; a variety of approaches to spread and scale; measurement strategies and effectiveness; and increasing the focus on spread and scale in population health (Wizemann and Thompson 2015b, 3).

Spread is an important concept in this report, which emphasizes reaching out to the population that needs the information or services. Scale focuses on investment, costs, and providing services to more people over time with less cost. Scaling is difficult to accomplish in health care. Sustainability is about persistence and commitment. Elements that health professionals can use to improve spread and scale are: assisting in the spread, scale, and sustainability of big data and monitoring techniques; registration such as registering people for health services; health marketing; early detection; incentives; and business medical models that make the most of efficiency and collaboration. The six drivers of population health improvement are metrics, resources, policy, research, relationships, and communication, all of which are discussed in this report.

Collaboration between Health Care and Public Health: Workshop Summary (2016)

Collaboration is a critical factor in the interface between health care and public health. Today, it is an important aspect of understanding health care. To explain the complexity, this report provides an example: "It is not possible to talk about advancing payment reform without discussing how to finance the change, improving asthma outcomes without discussing social determinants of health, or improving high blood pressure rates without looking at the infrastructure for healthy activities" (HMD 2016b, 3). After examining a variety of examples of successful collaboration between health care and public health, the report identified many common themes, such as building on success, leadership, data and metrics, setting clear goals and planning with effective implementation, innovation, sharing, and working with others (HMD 2016b). These themes apply to any collaborative effort in health care management and practice.

A Framework for Educating Health Professionals to Address the Social Determinants of Health (2016)

The World Health Organization (WHO) defines social determinants of health as "the conditions in which people are born, grow, work, live, and age, and the wider set of forces and systems shaping the conditions of daily life" (WHO 2016a). This report focuses on the importance of these determinants to health and what we need to do to better ensure that health care professionals are prepared to address these needs. Understanding the effects of these determinants should be part of academic programs and lifelong learning for health care professionals. The report provides a model that focuses on three domains: what should be done in education, by organizations, and the community (HMD 2016c, 7). The domains interact and each has its own strategies; for example, education uses experiential learning, collaborative learning, integrated curriculum, and continuing professional development. This report and its content are important to nursing education and particularly to community and public health content and clinical experiences.

The Research and Evidence-Based Practice Reports

Early on in the HMD's efforts to examine the status of health care delivery, there was recognition the importance of research and EBP. Utilization of EBP is identified as one of the five core health care profession competencies. More current reports expanded on the examination of EBP and its application in clinical practice. All of these reports are excellent resources for undergraduate and graduate faculty and students.

Knowing What Works in Health Care: A Roadmap for the Nation (2008)

As quality care is examined there is emphasis on EBP and the need to define diagnostic, treatment, and prevention services—how they work and under what conditions. Another important issue is how different health care providers handle specific problems. Cost is yet another factor in clinical decisions and should be considered, particularly as it relates to best practice. Quality is integral to all of these concerns and EBP. The report indicates that more must be done to support use of EBP: "The nation must significantly expand its capacity to use scientific evidence to assess 'what works' in health care. This report recommends an organizational framework for a national clinical effectiveness assessment program" (Eden 2008, 1). Effective evidence is described as knowledge that is explicit, systematic, and replicable, and it must be related to the real world. The major health policy challenges related to this recommendation are as follows (3, 5):

- **Constraining health care costs.** This can make a difference in reducing health care costs, but it can also limit care and quality.
- **Reducing geographic variation in the use of health care services.** There are uncertainties about what works and for whom.
- **Improving quality.** We need evidence to define quality care.
- **Empowering health care consumers.** Consumers and patients should be managers of their own health and health care and they require information in order to be empowered to make their decisions.
- **Making health coverage decisions.** All types of insurance plans are struggling with the challenges of learning how their covered populations might benefit from or be harmed by the newly available health services.

This report is a good EBP resource; it includes information about EBP and systematic reviews.

Learning What Works: Infrastructure Required for Comparative Effectiveness Research: Workshop Summary (2011)

With a goal of ensuring that 90 percent of clinical decisions will be supported by accurate, timely, and up-to-date evidence by 2020, the report *Learning What Works* addresses some of the issues that are important in reaching this goal (Olson, Grossmann, and McGinnis 2011). The purpose of this report is to examine the infrastructure that we need to support development of and access to comparative effectiveness information. This infrastructure includes staff with competencies related to comparative effectiveness research (CER) and HIT, information networks, communication, and coordination. The content includes an examination of the need for and value of CER, necessary actions, required information networks and expertise, and implementation priorities. We need more trials and studies, systematic reviews, innovative research strategies, and clinical registries to better synthesize what is learned from research into practice. CER assists in improving the effectiveness and value of health care. Effectiveness is a critical element that must be considered when research results are evaluated. The important themes relate to effective and efficient care, coordination and standards, moving from testing to practice, infrastructure to support CER, utilization of technological innovations, investment in HIT, a trained workforce, and the integration of public and private efforts (Olson, Grossmann, and McGinnis 2011, 14). As was mandated in the ACA, CER would have been part of the initiative to transform health care in the United States, and today it is included.

This report also comments on transforming health professions education, highlighting previous *Quality Chasm* reports on health professions education that emphasize a patient-centered health management focus, particularly noting the need for interprofessional teams, from early education through lifelong learning. Interprofessional issues have increased and now are more important. The Interprofessional Education Collaborative (IPEC), consisting of the AACN, the American Association of Colleges of Osteopathic Medicine (AACOM), the Association of Schools and Programs of Public Health (ASPPH), the American Association of Colleges of Pharmacy (AACP), the American Dental Education Association (ADEA), and the American Association of Medical Colleges (AAMC), developed core competencies that should underpin collaborative practice and thus affect interprofessional education at the academic level and interprofessional continuing education (IPEC 2011), discussed in more detail in chapter 4.

Finding What Works in Health Care: Standards for Systematic Reviews (2011)

Finding What Works focuses on research and EBP from the perspective of published systematic reviews (SR) of CER (Eden et al. 2011). The SR is the most effective tool for ensuring greater application of research in practice, although clearly just having a process to develop and share systematic reviews does not mean that practitioners will apply them.

Health care organizations are expected to have standards, which may be standards they create or borrow from external sources. These standards are guides for performance expectations and accountability. Standards are also needed to describe what is expected of SR development in order to allow for more effective identification, selection, and interpretation of evidence to support best practices. SRs provide evidence for clinical practice guidelines and thus have a major impact on clinical decisions. SRs focus on CER, which is "the generation and synthesis of evidence that compares the benefits and harms of alternative methods to prevent, diagnose, treat, and monitor a clinical condition or to improve the delivery of care" (Eden et al. 2011, 42). CER is used to better ensure effective, informed decision-making in the health care delivery system. Thus, there is a critical linkage of CER, SRs, and clinical practice guidelines. This report contains important content for research and EBP. In 2016, there was concern expressed about the growth of SRs and their value, for example, the influence of funders such as drug companies on the results of SRs (Harris 2016). We need better disclosure of the financial interests of authors of SRs to ensure that we are using best evidence without bias.

Clinical Practice Guidelines We Can Trust (2011)
Clinical practice guidelines (CPGs) are readily available today. The AHRQ has a large database of CPGs (more than 2,700) available through its National Guideline Clearinghouse (http://www.guideline.gov). There are also other sources of guidelines, and even with all the CPGs we have, we need to continue to develop them, particularly effective CPGs based on strong evidence: "CPGs provide opportunity to reduce inappropriate practice variation, enhance translation of research into practice, improve health care quality and safety, and influence the development of physician and hospital performance measures" (Graham 2011, xi). We not only need to have and apply CPGs, we also need to use them to collect data and measure quality.

With the proliferation of research, most practitioners do not have the time or expertise to sift through results to find data that can have an impact on their clinical decisions. Evidence-based CPGs provide a way to increase EBP; however, the quality of the CPGs must also be considered. For example, reviews should be done of the quality of the studies, their transparency, their use of effective expert groups, their use of preexisting guidelines, and any conflicts of interest.

The report *Knowing What Works in Health Care* alerted the HHS to the need for a public-private program that would "develop or endorse and promote standards that address the structure, process, reporting, and final products of systematic reviews of comparative effectiveness research and evidence-based clinical practice guidelines" (Eden 2008, 3). Clinical practice guidelines provide recommendations for health care providers based on best evidence to provide quality care, utilizing systematic reviews of evidence, particularly research. CPGs should describe clinical options in a clear manner and be reviewed routinely to determine if revisions are required based on current evidence.

This report includes additional content on CPGs and the need to use them effectively. It is an important resource for students, faculty, and nurses on the topic of CPGs, which nurses as well as physicians should apply.

Sharing Clinical Trial Data: Maximizing Benefits, Minimizing Risk (2015)

It is natural to accept that sharing clinical trial data is important to society and to patients. For participants, it confirms the value of their taking a risk for others. However, clinical trial data are not always shared, which is critical to other researchers who might use the results for additional research. In addition, limiting access limits the ability of other researchers to confirm or dispute results, and there have been situations where original results were not confirmed and later found to be invalid or incomplete (HMD 2015b).

There are difficulties with sharing data. A key one is privacy; participants expect that their individual information will be kept private and that it will be shared in a responsible manner. There may also be issues with intellectual property and commercial concerns related to the study results or methods used.

Key stakeholders (research funders, researchers, research participants, disease advocacy organizations, regulatory and oversight organizations and agencies, research ethics committees (institutional review boards [IRBs], research institutions and universities, and professional journals and organizations) need to engage in a culture of sharing. The report discusses the types of data, such as summary results or raw data, that might be shared and the risks and benefits attached to sharing each type. The conclusion is that there should be a culture of responsible sharing of clinical trial data with effective incentives to do so.

Health Care Informatics

Health care informatics technology became a part of the reports on health care, and today, this topic is even more relevant as HIT has expanded, in both its capabilities and its applications in health care delivery. There is greater need now for evaluation and also increased concern about ethics, fraud, and improved access to information to support QI efforts.

Health Literacy, eHealth, and Communication: Putting the Consumer First: Workshop Summary (2009)

With the growing need to improve the quality of care, a study done in 2006 surveyed health care opinion leaders to rate the effectiveness of a variety of strategies to improve care (Shea, Shih, and Davis 2007). The results indicated that 67 percent thought accelerating the development and use of HIT was important. Health informatics is viewed as a method for improving quality, safety, and efficiency (Hernandez 2009). Today, EMRs, EHRs, and personal health records (PHRs) are critical elements of HIT. This should provide greater health information exchange; however, interoperability has become a critical concern in developing effective and efficient systems. EMR adoption rates are still improving. Health information exchange should include not only hospitals but also other types of health care providers, individuals, and HCOs, including medical practices and clinics.

Consumers also use electronic systems to obtain personal health information. The rate of consumer Internet use to find health information has increased since the publication of this 2009 report. Consumers are looking for information to guide their decisions. The critical factors in the ability to access this electronic information are access to and ability to use technology and the Internet and English proficiency. Greater use of information and greater availability of effective and reliable information can help patients prepare for a medical appointment if they understand the information. This report provides many examples of ehealth strategies and their impacts on different populations, with a focus on the patient and consumer.

Health IT and Patient Safety: Building Safer Systems for Better Care (2011)

Health IT has an impact on the ease of documentation and thus affects the quality of care and number of errors. As noted in this report, HIT should maximize patient safety and minimize harm, but research findings are mixed on whether or not HIT actually succeeds at these aims. Why do we not have better evidence? HIT-related safety data are lacking because of the lack of clear standards of measurement or a repository of data that can be analyzed and used to improve. The ability to share information and build this repository is also limited by legal and ethical issues such as nondisclosure and confidentiality requirements that interfere with sharing information about adverse events associated with HIT (IOM 2011b). Since the publication of this report, more has been done at the national level to develop more effective measurements of effectiveness. Along with HIT that involves the health care provider, another area of development is the use of information technology by patients and families, for example, monitoring their health electronically, accessing personal health records, and using a variety of mobile applications related to health.

Today, there is greater use of EMRs in physician offices, clinics, home health, hospitals, and other health care settings. The ACA supported greater use of EMRs in all health care settings. However, just using HIT does not guarantee that care will always be high-quality and error-free. We need standards, funding, demonstration projects, and increased monitoring of health care outcomes in order to develop effective use of HIT in the United States.

Vital Signs: Core Metrics for Health and Health Care Progress (2015)
As more emphasis has been placed on the serious problem of quality care there have been greater efforts made to assess and address the problems. This is a good thing, but also means an expansion of measures. As noted in this report, we have many measures now to assess care, but many lack focus and consistency and may not lend themselves to effective organization of data obtained. This all impacts how effective these measures actually are at improving care. Measures need to be streamlined to provide more effective benchmarks for assessing progress and focusing on high-priority areas. This discussion about core metrics includes healthy people, care quality, lower costs, and engaged people. The report provides important information to better understand the complex area of health care metrics and quality care. See the report's recommendations for a core measure set with priority measures related to issues like life expectancy, overweight and obesity, preventive services, access to care, and others (Blumenthal, Malphrus, and McGinnis 2015, 15–16).

It is important to note that collecting data on these measures will be a complex process with additional burdens for providers, HCOs, and the entire health care delivery system. In the end, effective implementation of the core measures by stakeholders will be influenced by each measure's relevance, reliability, and utility. Standardized measures should improve evaluation efficiency and effectiveness.

Nursing
Nursing is an important topic in the reports, and some reports focus on nursing, as described below, and others apply indirectly to nursing due to the importance of nurses and nursing care in the health care delivery system. In addition, all of the focus concerns for the reports relate either directly or indirectly to nursing. This section focuses on the reports that specifically address nursing.

Keeping Patients Safe: Transforming the Work Environment for Nurses (2004)
Although germane to nursing in any health care setting, *Keeping Patients Safe* focuses on acute care. It addresses critical quality and safety issues

with an emphasis on nursing care and nurses, particularly in the work environment. As the report states, "When we are hospitalized, in a nursing home, or managing a chronic condition in our own homes—at some of our most vulnerable moments—nurses are the health care providers we are most likely to encounter, spend the greatest amount of time with, and be dependent upon for our recovery" (Child 2004, ix). Following a review of the clinical work environment, the report discusses design for a work environment in which nurses can provide safer, higher-quality patient care. It explores health care errors, patient safety risk factors, the central role of the nurse in patient safety, work environment threats to patient safety, and periods of time when there have been nursing shortages. Although this report was published in 2004, it is still very relevant to nursing and health care delivery today.

Similar to earlier quality reports, this report calls for a change from blaming individuals for errors to greater consideration of the many system factors that influence outcomes, for example, equipment failures, inadequate staff training, lack of clear supervision and direction, inadequate staffing levels, need for nursing leadership, and so on. Making the necessary improvements will require a transformation of the work environment and process. It is first important to understand how work is done so that patient safety measures can be integrated in the nursing work environment. The report identifies several major concerns related to direct care in nursing, such as the need to monitor patients (*surveillance*, defined as the "purposeful and ongoing acquisition, interpretation, and synthesis of patient data for clinical decision-making" [McCloskey and Bulechek 2000, 629]), the need for nursing interventions that meet patients' physiological needs and help patients and families with loss (such as complete loss of or limited function) and emotional needs, the need for better patient and family education, and the need to coordinate care and work collaboratively with interprofessional teams (Child 2004). Since the publication of this report there is now more emphasis placed on coordination, collaboration, and interprofessional teams.

The report recommends (1) adopting transformational leadership and evidence-based management (EBM), (2) maximizing the capability of the workforce, and (3) creating and sustaining cultures of safety. The report's recommendations highlight the need for transformational leadership, a culture of safety, interprofessional teamwork, staff education, staffing levels that meet needs, and greater understanding of safety and interventions to ensure quality. The four key topics discussed in *Keeping Patients Safe* are

(1) work design, (2) safety and the central role of the nurse in ensuring safety, (3) quality, and (4) nursing shortages (Child 2004).

Leadership is important in making these changes. This topic should be integrated throughout the curriculum, at both the undergraduate and graduate levels, by focusing on the role of leadership in quality improvement. This is a landmark report for nursing; it contains important material for nursing education, staff education, nursing management, direct care nursing, and nursing research.

The Future of Nursing: Leading Change, Advancing Health (2011)

This landmark report on nursing is based on the previous work described in other *Quality Chasm* reports. One of its key messages is that nurses should assume new and expanded roles in a redesigned health care system—but to do this, there must be greater flexibility in practice supported by professional education and training. Thus, improving nursing education must also be part of this movement (IOM 2011a).

Utilizing forums held across the country, the committee of experts led discussions about transforming practice, education, and leadership. This report is the collection of the results from these forums. As the title indicates, nurses need to become leaders of the changes that are required to improve health care. The report makes eight important recommendations. How do the recommendations relate to changes needed in nursing education, the *Quality Chasm* reports, and the five health care professions core competencies? The eight recommendations are discussed below (IOM 2011a).

> **Recommendation 1: Remove scope-of-practice barriers.** The report focuses on the scope of practice for advanced practice registered nurses (APRNs) to ensure that they can practice to the full extent of their education. APRNs are just as responsible for quality care as any other health care provider. We need to ensure that APRN education programs integrate the five core health care profession competencies into the curriculum and contain sufficient content on quality improvement. APRNs need to understand the national, organizational, individual practice, and patient implications of quality. APRNs should be leaders in QI wherever they practice.
>
> **Recommendation 2: Expand opportunities for nurses to lead and diffuse collaborative improvement efforts.** We need greater opportunities for nurses to hold leadership positions in all types of HCOs, education, professional organizations, health policy and government, and so on. None of this will happen if nursing education continues to ignore QI in the curriculum or treat it as a minor subject. Latter parts

of this book discuss specific information that is critical to QI. If nurses are prepared, they will have greater opportunities to assume the lead in HCOs regarding care improvement. In addition, each nurse who provides care at the bedside should be the first line of defense for each patient.

Recommendation 3: Implement nurse residency programs. We have long advocated nurse residency programs, and we need support for this from accrediting bodies, government, HCOs, and state boards of nursing. These programs should include the five health care core competencies. The difficulty with this recommendation is finding funding for these programs. Until the funding problem is solved, most residencies will be funded by grants, and may or may not be continued after the grant cycle is completed if the HCO cannot afford to continue the program. Additional content about nurse residencies is found in chapter 4.

Recommendation 4: Increase the proportion of nurses with a baccalaureate degree to 80 percent by 2020. Increasing these numbers also requires funding. In addition, the increased number of expected nurse retirements has not yet happened—but it will. Recruitment of qualified students is of great concern. We cannot afford to waste time and energy on entering students who may not be successful or fully understand the expectations of the profession. We need to put greater effort in recruiting the right match for the job and finding out more about applicants before acceptance. We need greater ability to assess students at risk and provide program supports to assist these students and also recognize that some applicants should not be accepted or may have to be dropped from programs if they are not successful. We also need greater student and faculty diversity. At some point, we must make decisions about the graduates we are sending into practice.

Recommendation 5: Double the number of nurses with a doctorate by 2020. This recommendation may not be so easy to fulfill. We have the PhD in nursing, and now we have the Doctor of Nursing Practice (DNP) degree. The latter is a practice degree, not a research-oriented degree; however, we have found that faculty are enrolling in these programs, often with no intention of practicing, but rather to continue teaching. The DNP is not considered a doctorate by some universities, in the sense that persons with a DNP may not be given tenured positions (which are generally reserved for researchers), but rather clinical positions. It is unclear what the result will be. We will need to increase the percentage at a faster rate per year if we are to meet this goal.

Recommendation 6: Ensure that nurses engage in lifelong learning. Continuing education (CE) has long been a part of nursing, but in general it has not been considered worthy of much attention. Some states require CE for licensure renewal, but the route to CE is fairly easy. It is also difficult to prove that CE has had any impact on the quality of care. Recently, there has been some attempt to organize and recommend CE changes by focusing on an interprofessional approach. There is no guarantee that this will result in any additional positive impact on care. The typical way RNs get their CE is to go to a conference, but they can also earn the requisite CE credits through online modules, which certainly do not require any interprofessional interaction. Most nurses just do what is convenient, quick, and cheap. In many cases the content has nothing to do with what the nurses do in practice, and there is no requirement that the content be relevant to practice. This recommendation is important because improving competency should improve care, but determining if CE accomplishes this is difficult. Currently, routine participation in CE is a problem unless employers require CE, the state board of nursing requires CE for licensure renewal, or there are specialty requirements for CE. These are critical issues that must be addressed. Some nurse leaders have suggested we use demonstration and documentation of continued competence, which might be done through portfolio documentation of cases and skills the nurse has performed during the year or through simulated experiences. Additional information on CE in other reports is discussed in chapters 3 and 4.

Recommendation 7: Prepare and enable nurses to lead change to advance health. We must do much more, beginning at the under-graduate level and through graduate programs, to offer courses that engage students in the leadership development process and keep them in it for a lifetime. Schools of nursing need active integration of this type of content and experience in every course and need to devise methods that facilitate the expansion of learning about and developing leadership.

Recommendation 8: Build an infrastructure for the collection and analysis of interprofessional health care workforce data. The Workforce Commission and the HRSA should collaborate with state licensing boards, state nursing workforce centers, and the Department of Labor in this effort to ensure that the data are timely and publicly accessible. The ACA had mandated the establishment of this workforce commission; however, funding had been slow even before the 2017 challenges to the ACA. This has relevance for nursing education, as it will provide a resource for projections of need.

The Future of Nursing report is a rich source of information for faculty and for students, both undergraduate and graduate (IOM 2011a). Either sections of the report or the entire report can be assigned for examination and discussion. It has relevance for courses on such topics as transition or introduction to professional nursing, leadership and management, health policy, trends in health care and the profession, education, and research. All students should be aware of this report and its implications.

It is important to recognize that *The Future of Nursing* report is part of a series of reports on quality care. The critical reports that examine the problems in health care and set up a process for monitoring and improving care are the most important parts of this series. This report on nursing focuses primarily on regulation, degrees and number of nurses with certain degrees, and the need for nursing leadership in improving care. However, combining this report with the earlier reports makes *The Future of Nursing* even more relevant to the delivery of health care. As nurses, to focus only on this nursing report is to miss the major messages about the need for improvement, why we have this need, and how we can meet the need. An update report, which is critical to understanding the current status of the recommendations, has been published (Altman, Stith Butler, and Shern 2016) and is discussed later in this part.

Future Directions of Credentialing Research in Nursing: Workshop Summary (2015)

Nurses may be certified and also participate in credentialing programs, which reflect nursing standards and outcome measures, including training. It is assumed that certification and credentialing have a positive effect on practice and quality; however, there is not sufficient evidence to support this assumption. The ANCC partnered with the HMD on a workshop to examine this issue. Many other nursing organizations served as sponsors for this workshop. The following are the workshop topics (McCoy and Weisfeld 2015, 3):

- Emergent priorities for research in nursing credentialing
- Critical knowledge gaps and methodological limitations in the field
- Promising developments in research methodologies, health metrics, and data infrastructures to better evaluate the impact of nursing credentialing
- Short- and long-term strategies to encourage continued activity in nursing credentialing research

Based on the aims for the workshop, the presenters and attendees discuss the critical issues and identify themes or issues that need further consideration and action related to a shared research framework, improvement in data (collection, analysis, sharing, and so on), changing roles of nursing, need for credentialing research, and resources to support these efforts (HMD 2015b).

The Future of Home Health Care: Workshop Summary (2015)

This workshop and its report provide a review of the status of home health care in a health care delivery system that is moving more toward a community focus (Weisfeld and Lustig 2015). In addition, there is more interest in the role of home health care in supporting aging in place (home) and assisting high-risk adults (such as older adults) with chronic illnesses and disabilities in receiving health care and long-term services. The passage of the ACA also stimulated more interest in care in the home. It is noted that there now is a spectrum of home health care: informal services (the largest group), formal personal care services, Medicare skilled home health care, home-based primary care, and hospital at home (the smallest group). The report discusses the current state of home health care—issues and trends, the home health care workforce, models of care and payment, use of technology, and partnerships and collaborations with home health care services. Home health care is a critical work setting for nurses and one in which they should assume more leadership (Marrelli 2016).

Best Practices for Better Health Care

After addressing general concerns about health care quality, the HMD turned to best practices to discover and demonstrate effective approaches to improving care. The following reports focus on several examples of best practice and represent some of these reports that examine a variety of health and health care delivery issues and problems. The HMD website includes these reports and many other reports not included in this book (http://www.nationalacademies.org/hmd/Reports.aspx).

Preventing Childhood Obesity: Health in the Balance (2005)

The epidemic of childhood obesity is a critical pediatric health problem with long-term implications for adult health (Koplan, Liverman, and Kraak 2005). This report notes that obesity affects boys and girls in all areas of the country, across all socioeconomic strata, and across all ethnic groups, with African American, Hispanic, and Native American children experiencing a higher level of obesity.

Costs of obesity and incidence have increased since this report was published. The report identifies goals for obesity prevention in children and youth, both long term and intermediate, to guide health policymakers at the local, state, and federal levels, health care professionals, and health care organizations. Examples of intermediate goals focus on practical approaches such as walking to school, emphasizing the importance of play and exercise for children, and development of community recreational facilities.

Quality through Collaboration: The Future of Rural Health **(2005)**

Quality through Collaboration (IOM 2005) addresses the critical quality care issues of populations in rural areas, which represent an estimated 20 percent of the US population. These diverse populations are found in all regions of the country, and represent vulnerable health care populations. Rural areas have the same health care quality challenges as other areas, but they also face some circumstances that make it more difficult to achieve quality care. Some major health care services may not be provided or may be limited, such as emergency medical services, mental health and substance abuse services, and oral health care. There are shortages of health care providers and specialists in many areas of the country, but the deficits (both generally and in specialty providers) in rural areas are greater in overall number.

Rural populations tend to be older than urban populations and experience higher rates of limitations in daily activities as a result of chronic conditions. Compared to urban areas, rural populations typically have more health problems and poorer health behaviors, such as smoking, obesity, and less regular exercise (IOM 2005). We need to improve data collection about health in rural areas, compile evidence to improve care in rural areas, increase education about EBP, and formulate quality improvement measures for rural areas. The five health care professions core competencies apply to care in rural areas, and they should be viewed from the perspective of rural health care needs. There is no doubt that we need more rural health care providers and HCOs to reduce travel time to provide appropriate, affordable, and effective health care across the life span—in essence, to make quality care more accessible in rural areas. Both personal and population health programs are essential to improving health.

The Federal Office of Rural Health Policy (FORHP) is a part of the Health Resources and Services Administration (HRSA) under the HHS. It promotes better health care service in rural areas. Its website describes FORHP activities (http://www.hrsa.gov/ruralhealth/). This report is particularly relevant to schools of nursing located in rural areas or using clinical agencies in rural areas, although all nursing students need to understand US rural health care needs.

*Improving the Quality of Health Care for Mental
and Substance-Use Conditions* **(2006)**

The need for mental health and substance-use services is high, although treatment and services have slowly improved. These problems impact many people in all areas of the United States. Based on 2006 data, mental and substance-use conditions are the leading cause of combined disability and death among women and second highest among men (IOM 2006b). We need to ensure that the health care system provides care for these vulnerable populations, recognizes patient preferences, needs, and values so that it is patient-centered; improves care equity with no discrimination due to their medical problems or for any other reason; applies coordination, EBP, and effective use of HIT to ensure quality care; provides sufficient reimbursement methods; and develops research to meet the needs of these populations.

We have effective treatments for many mental health problems, but these services have to be made accessible and affordable. Some mental health problems require long-term care, and this care also must be accessible, effective, and affordable. In addition, we need to deal with the persistent issue of stigma. There has been greater emphasis on research that examines the interplay between genetic, environmental, biologic, and psychosocial factors in brain function, but much more remains to be done. Mental health and substance-abuse care is not always at the level it should be, and poor care can lead to more serious problems. Mental health needs are frequently associated with other medical conditions; for example, people hospitalized with a myocardial infarction are found to also have a greater risk (one in five) for major depression. Substance abuse leads to multiple biological illnesses, to mental illness, and to sociological problems (abuse, violence, crime, loss of job, limited education, divorce, single parenting, housing issues, and more). This care must meet all of the requirements for quality care as addressed in the *Quality Chasm* series, such as the six aims of high-quality health care (STEEEP). This report is a valuable resource for psychiatric-mental health (behavioral) content and clinical experiences. Later content discusses the increase in opioid addiction in the United States and its impact on public health.

From Cancer Patient to Cancer Survivor: Lost in Transition (2006)

In the past cancer care concentrated mostly on acute care, but now many patients are living longer with cancer. Care for survivors who now are considered to have a chronic illness becomes even more important. This requires new approaches to help the more than ten million American cancer survivors. Cancer survivors need coordinated care, and this becomes particularly important when they transition from active cancer treatment to long-term care where follow-up is critical. The aims of the report are to (Hewitt and Ganz 2006, 2):

- Raise awareness of the medical, functional, and psychosocial consequences of cancer and its treatment;
- Define quality health care for cancer survivors and identify strategies to achieve it; and
- Improve the quality of life of cancer survivors.

The focus is on cancer survivorship, which is a "distinct phase of the cancer trajectory which has been relatively neglected in advocacy, education, clinical practice, and research" (Hewitt and Ganz 2006, 2). The report discusses the essential components of survivorship care. It offers a different perspective on cancer care that is very important to include in content and clinical experiences.

Cancer Care for the Whole Patient: Meeting Psychosocial Health Needs (2007)

Cancer Care for the Whole Patient: Meeting Psychosocial Health Needs (Adler and Page 2007) expands the examination of cancer. It recommends that all parties that establish or use standards for the quality of cancer care adopt the following as a guideline: All cancer care should ensure the provision of appropriate psychosocial health services by methods such as effective communication between patients and providers, meeting psychosocial needs, and using effective planning including follow-up and changes as need.

This report and its recommendations provide excellent examples of psychosocial interventions. Some schools of nursing are reducing mental health content, but this ignores the importance of understanding the needs and care for patients in multiple situations that require psychosocial support.

Emergency Medical Services at the Crossroads (2006)

Emergency medical services (EMS) "encompass the initial stages of the emergency care continuum. It includes emergency calls to 911; dispatch of emergency personnel to the scene of an illness or trauma; and triage, treatment, and transport of patients by ambulance and air medical service" (IOM 2006a, 1). Effective emergency treatment must consider timing of care and the quality of the services as both cam impact patient outcomes. This report notes that the current delivery system has some major weaknesses: insufficient coordination, disparities in response times, variable quality of care, lack of readiness for disasters, health care professional identity issues in emergency services, and limited use of EBP. The report discusses needs and strategies for improvement.

Hospital-Based Emergency Care: At the Breaking Point (2007)

The emergency care system is described as "overburdened, underfunded, and highly fragmented" (IOM 2007c, 1). The report points out that emergency departments (EDs) may not be able to routinely handle the load and must then send patients to other hospitals. It also notes that the disaster response system needs improvement. This report is one of a series of reports on emergency care that includes *Emergency Care for Children: Growing Pains* (IOM 2007a), *Emergency Medical Services at the Crossroads* (IOM 2006a), and a follow-up workshop, *Future of Emergency Care in the United States Health System* (IOM 2007b). *Hospital-Based Emergency Care: At the Breaking Point* concentrates on the impact of EDs on hospitals and the broader health care delivery system; patient flow; HIT; ED workforce needs and problems; quality care; and ED research (IOM 2007c). The report also comments on the challenges of providing emergency care in rural settings such as lack of hospitals or hospitals with EMS, ambulance services, and distance often required to receive this needed care.

Emergency Care for Children: Growing Pains (2007)

Children who receive emergency medical services have unique medical needs, and the family has a major role in pediatric emergency care. Physiological differences from adults, safety, the higher risk for errors in treating children, and special communication needs are all matters of concern. As noted in this report and other related reports, the emergency and trauma care system needs improvement. It is fragmented and lacks coordination among the various providers and follow-up services. Use of emergency care has increased, although some areas have had changes in their access to these services with some services closing or merging. Ambulance diversion is common in some areas due to the volume of patients, and this impacts the quality of EMS (IOM 2007a). This report is a good resource for students studying pediatric care and for staff who provide pediatric emergency services. It focuses on the role of pediatric emergency services as an integrated component of the overall health system; system-wide pediatric emergency care planning, preparedness, coordination; EMS funding; pediatric training in professional education; and research in pediatric emergency care.

Future of Emergency Care (2007)

Unlike the other reports, this is a summary of a series of workshops held across the United States to discuss the other three EMS reports: *Emergency Medical Services at the Crossroads* (IOM, 2006a), *Hospital-Based Emergency Care: At the Breaking Point* (IOM, 2007c), and *Emergency Care for Children: Growing Pains* (IOM, 2007a). The emergency system is a critical part of the health care system, and as these reports on emergency care show, there are multiple problems, for example, overcrowding, lack of coordination, workforce shortages, variability in the quality of care, lack of effective disaster preparedness, limited research to support EBP, and limited services for children requiring emergency care (IOM 2007b). Throughout the reports on EMS, similar concerns are identified and discussed—supporting the consensus that there are consistent issues that need to be addressed.

Preterm Birth: Causes, Consequences, and Prevention (2007)

This report examines the problem of preterm births in the United States. The number of preterm births has increased, and the increase is more marked in some areas of the country than others. This health problem is connected to racial, ethnic, and socioeconomic disparities. Preterm births increase the risk of mortality and short- and long-term health and development problems and may lead to many different complications. There are also serious implications for the families as well as economic costs (Behrman and Stith Butler 2007). We need to know much more about the causes of preterm births and what can be done to prevent them. This report describes preterm birth priority areas and issues such as increased interprofessional research, disparities, improved care for infants and mothers, and a better understanding of causes and prevention. This report is a good resource for maternal-child, public, and community health providers and facilities, and policymakers at local, state, and national levels, as it identifies practice concerns, issues for research consideration, and areas of improvement to achieve better outcomes.

Retooling for an Aging America: Building the Healthcare Workforce (2008)

This report focuses on the needs of the older vulnerable population (IOM 2008). With seniors (those sixty-five years of age and older) constituting approximately 20 percent of the population and the long-term expectation that this population will increase, they are a critical concern for health care services. Medical care has enabled people to live longer. Many are in relatively good health, though chronic illness is a problem. Patients over the age of seventy-five average three chronic conditions and may take four or more medications.

The health care workforce is unprepared for this population with its complex needs, and half of the providers for this population, such as nurse aides, receive very low pay. Of older adults who receive care in the home, 90 percent get additional help from family and friends, and 80 percent rely solely on family and friends for care. The report identifies three initiatives to address this problem: (1) focus on changing and improving roles and responsibilities of health care workers with consideration given to education and training; (2) increase understanding of the needs of this population and their family and friends; and (3) develop new approaches and models to improve care for older adults across the continuum of care, including reimbursement.

Schools of nursing are expanding content on the older population, but much more is needed, along with increased clinical experience with this population. Much more is required to improve care for this growing, vulnerable population. The John A. Hartford Foundation is an excellent resource for addressing nursing for this population. Its mission is to shape the quality of health care of older adults through nursing excellence and it emphasizes the values of interdisciplinary and interprofessional approaches, quality care, knowledge, and respect for older adults and the people who care for them (http://www.johnahartford.org/about).

Relieving Pain in America: A Blueprint for Transforming Prevention, Care, Education, and Research (2011)

Due to Section 4305 of the ACA, the HHS requested that the HMD examine pain management, recognizing pain as a major public health problem. Pain management is part of patient-centered care, impacts many areas of health care, and is a universal experience. The report notes that at the time the report was published, common chronic pain conditions affected at least 116 million US adults, at a cost of $560–$635 billion annually in direct medical treatment costs and lost productivity" (IOM 2011d, 1). The 2012 National Health Interview Survey (NHIS) found that "an estimated 25.3 million adults (11.2 percent) experience daily pain—that is, they had pain every day for the 3 months prior to the survey. In addition, nearly 40 million adults (17.6 percent) experience severe levels of pain and are also likely to have worse health status" (NCCIH 2015).

This *Quality Chasm* report recognizes that pain is complex and influenced by biological, behavioral, environmental, and societal factors. Understanding pain requires more knowledge about its neurological and genetic aspects. There is a need for new tools and metrics to better diagnose and measure pain and then develop more effective interventions. The report explores the meaning of pain, risks for pain, impact of pain, types of pain and causes, and cultural issues. Pain is viewed as a public health challenge that includes consideration of diversity, disparities, and cost. Treatment, education about pain, and research on pain are all examined in the report.

The report concludes with a blueprint for transforming pain prevention, care, education, and research and identifies who should be involved in meeting the goals, such as the HHS, the AHRQ, and so on (Table 6-1, IOM 2011d, 272–75). We need to improve assessment and treatment of pain, and this blueprint provides some guidance.

In 2016, with the growing substance abuse problem across the United States, effective pain management must be a priority. The opioid epidemic and its impact on care delivery and health is discussed more in chapter 4. Pain management is a critical element of nursing care, and nursing education should include more on this problem in all types of programs and degrees. This report provides an overview of the problem and describes recommendations or strategies to improve pain management for patients.

Dying in America: Improving Quality and Honoring Individual Preferences Near the End of Life (2014)

"Healthcare delivery for people nearing the end of life has changed significantly in the past two decades" (IOM 2014, 1). We have experienced many changes that impact this experience, such as increased number of older Americans, access problems for some who need care (related to problems with reimbursement, transportation, availability of specialty care, etc.), and the fragmented health care system first described in the initial *Quality Chasm* reports. Can we improve this care for the dying patient? One intervention is to improve patient understanding of dying and their choices, including use of advanced planning and shared decision-making, which are included in ACA provisions. We also need to develop better measurement of care for the dying patient. Dying involves the need to provide social, psychological, and spiritual support with a patient-centered and, if the patient agrees, family-centered approach. Palliative care offers patients the option to maintain the highest quality of life possible. We need to know more about palliative care and its use across the continuum of care, and not just for the dying patient. This report examines these issues including education of health care professionals to better prepare them to address the needs of the dying patient. We can improve this care for many people and engage the patient in the process so that individual preferences are considered. In the long term, this should have a positive impact on meeting individual needs, improving care, and reducing health care costs. Nurses are directly involved in this care and should assume leadership in ensuring quality care for dying patients and their families.

Another concern discussed in this report is the fact that more than one quarter of adults seventy-five and older have not thought much about their view of their end of life. The report provides a description of the core components for a proposed quality end of life (see Table S-1, IOM 2014, 8–9). The report content includes a variety of topics such as patient- and family-centered care, comprehensive care, clinician-patient communication and advanced care planning, professional education and development, policies and reimbursement for this care, and public education and engagement.

Improving Diagnosis in Health Care (2015)

This report focuses on an important type of error that is not often discussed. A diagnostic error is "the failure to (a) establish an accurate and timely explanation of the patient's problem(s) or (b) communicate that explanation to the patient" (Balogh, Miller, and Call 2015, xi). Timeliness and accuracy are critical elements of diagnosis. Overdiagnosis can lead to many problems and increase costs, impacting quality, but it is often not considered to be an error and thus is difficult to identify per patient. Failures in the diagnostic process that do not lead to errors are designated as near misses. Data on this error are limited due to the use of few reliable tracking measures. Often when errors in diagnosis are identified, they are identified retrospectively. This is not a minor problem: Annually, 5 percent of US adults receiving outpatient care experience a diagnostic error (Balogh, Miller, and Call 2015). Patients are a critical element in catching this type of error. Another critical element in catching diagnostic errors is interprofessional collaboration. In addition to these issues, other concerns are identified and require improvement, such as staff training, effective use of clinical reasoning, teamwork and integration of different professionals such as radiology and pathology, communication, effective use of HIT in the diagnostic process, measurement of these errors, and the need for a culture of safety that allows staff to be open about diagnostic concerns and errors (Balogh, Miller, and Call 2015).

Other issues mentioned in the report that require more examination are the impacts of payment systems and medical liability on the diagnostic process and public reporting and accountability. The report provides a detailed examination of a topic that is not usually addressed. Recommendations for improvement focus on the areas noted above.

Opportunities to Promote Children's Behavioral Health: Health Care Reform and Beyond Workshop Summary (2015)

The ACA has provisions that may increase care access for children with behavioral health needs. These provisions require many insurance plans to provide prevention, treatment, and rehabilitation for mental health and substance abuse disorders for children. This report discusses these opportunities and how they may improve the quality of care for children and assist parents in coping with behavioral health issues with their children (Olson and Keren 2015). It examines multiple factors including community health centers, school-based health care services, home visiting programs, social services and child welfare, early childhood education, and schools. This report is relevant to psychiatric-mental health care, pediatrics, and public and community health.

Psychosocial Interventions for Mental and Substance-Abuse Disorders: A Framework for Establishing Evidence-Based Standards (2015)

The report notes that approximately 20 percent of Americans have mental health and substance use disorders that impact their morbidity and mortality (England, Stith Butler, and Gonzalez 2015). We have a gap in what is known about these disorders, treatment, and care received. The ACA provisions might have had an impact on improving this care and thus the health of those with these needs. There is a need for greater accountability and performance measurement. The report notes that it is necessary to develop a framework for establishing standards for psychosocial interventions. The key findings from the examination of this problem indicate that mental health and substance use disorders are serious public health problems; that there are a variety of psychosocial interventions that may have a positive impact these disorders; and that some of the effective interventions (based on research) are not used routinely.

Strategies to Improve Cardiac Arrest Survival: A Time to Act (2015)

Since time is critical when a cardiac arrest occurs, delayed action is an important issue to understand. It is necessary to identify effective steps that can be taken to reduce the problem and reduce mortality or complications of long-term chronic health problems. We need more data about resuscitation (incidence, treatment), which requires more effective measurement (Graham, McCoy, and Schultz 2015). The report discusses the chain of survival model (early access, early CPR, early defibrillation, early ACLS, early post-resuscitative care) that has been applied since 1991. This is an area of health care that requires the engagement of multiple health care providers, organizations, communities, and all levels of government. The report's proposed framework focuses on six steps: "Comprehensive surveillance and reporting; community engagement; new treatments and treatment paradigms, training and education; local translation of research into practice; and continuous quality improvement" (Graham, McCoy, and Schultz 2015, 8). Leadership, accountability, and transparency should be integrated throughout the initiative. We need greater data collection and dissemination of information; for example, it is recommended that the CDC establish a National Cardiac Arrest Registry. Local and state governments need to collaborate with the federal government to collect data. The public needs greater public awareness and training in responding to cardiac arrests. Care by health care professionals needs to be improved in all settings—from emergency responders through acute care and postcare. Research needs to be expanded to increase understanding of cardiac arrests and treatment. None of this can be accomplished without stakeholder collaboration.

Obesity in the Early Childhood Years: State of the Science and Implementation of Promising Solutions: Workshop in Brief (2016)

This report expands on work in the 2005 report on childhood obesity. Early childhood (from birth to age five) is considered a crucial time period for reducing obesity in the United States. Eating patterns are established early, and parents with children in this age group are more inclined to respond to information about this problem (Olson 2016). The report describes obesity prevalence and trends. Other related topics covered in the report are epigenetics, food, modifiable protective and risk factors, effective interventions, and partnerships with multiple stakeholders to develop and implement interventions. Given the critical level of obesity in children and adults in the United States, this report provides important information for health care providers in all settings, including public and community health, school health, and so on.

Preventing Bullying through Science, Policy, and Practice (2016)

Bullying is a longtime problem, but one that has increased, particularly due to digital access (Rivara and Le Menestrel 2016). The CDC defines bullying as "any unwanted aggressive behavior(s) by another youth or group of youths who are not siblings or current dating partners that involves an observed or perceived power imbalance and is repeated multiple times or is highly likely to be repeated. Bullying may inflict harm or distress on the targeted youth including physical, psychological, social, or educational harm" (CDC 2016a). This definition is used in this report. Definitions and ineffective measurement are barriers to fully appreciating the level of the problem. The report notes that cyber bullying should not be separated from bullying as the factors related to both, including the negative consequences and interventions, are similar or the same. It is critical that bullying not be viewed as a normal part of growing up, though it typically is seen this way. It may lead to major health problems such as anxiety, depression, and substance abuse. Suicide has also occurred in response to bullying. Individual reactions to it may be short- and long-term, carried into adulthood. The children and youth who do the bullying also have major problems such as depression, participation in high-risk behaviors, difficulty socializing with peers, and so on.

Prevention, as well as active interventions when bullying occurs, is critical for all communities, as discussed in this report. This requires multiple types of interventions and the involvement of multiple stakeholders, such as children and youth, parents (individuals and groups such as Parent Teacher Associations), educators, health care providers, social services, law enforcement, local government and services, and so on. Research shows that some policies and programs are helpful. Applying these results is important.

A National Trauma Care System: Integrating Military and Civilian Trauma Systems to Achieve Zero Preventable Deaths after Injury (2016)

"Trauma care in the military and civilian sectors is a portrait of contradiction—lethal contradiction. On one hand, the nation has never seen better systems of care for those wounded on the battlefield or severely injured in the United States. On the other hand, many trauma patients, depending on when and where they are injured, do not receive the benefit of those gains. Far too many needlessly die or sustain lifelong disabilities as a result" (Berwick, Downey, and Cornett 2016, xxxvii). Military trauma care has improved and expanded over the years, though it is not perfect; can it be used to develop more and better civilian services? The key elements are identified in the report from both a military and a civilian perspective (Table S-1, Berwick, Downey, and Cornett 2016, 11–14).

Health Care Professions Education

This section discusses reports that focus on health care professions education. They are discussed providing a review of the status of health care professions education and need for changes.

Health Professions Education (2003)

Education of health professionals is viewed as a bridge to quality care. The discussion in the IOM report *Health Professions Education: A Bridge to Quality* (Greiner and Knebel 2003) centers on the need to have qualified, competent staff to improve health care and concludes that all health professions education should change to meet the growing demands of current and future health care systems. The report clearly states that the goal of health professions education should be outcome-based education. Health care in the United States requires changes to improve health care quality, and these changes require an increase in content and experiences focused on quality improvement.

These recommendations are hardly surprising. The report, however, makes it clear that health professions education has not kept current with health care needs, EBP, HIT, technology, diversity changes, and leadership requirements— shortcomings that put health care profession education even further behind in light of newer recommendations. *The Essentials of Baccalaureate Education for Professional Nursing Practice* reflects the importance of all of the health care professions core competencies: "Yet the current challenges before us are twofold: to determine why the current workforce of baccalaureate-prepared nurses is not fully actualizing the [HMD] core competencies and to consider ways to strengthen nursing curricula to better educate nurses" (AACN 2008b, 259–60). The five core competencies recommended for implementation by all organizations involved in the education of health care professionals are as follows (Greiner and Knebel 2003, 49–63):

- **Provide patient-centered care.** Focus on the patient rather than the disease or the clinician.
- **Work in interprofessional teams.** Use the best health care professionals for the needs of the patient and work together to accomplish effective patient care outcomes.
- **Employ evidence-based practice.** Integrate best research results, clinical expertise, and patient values to make patient care decisions.
- **Apply quality improvement.** Use effective measurement and interventions to improve.
- **Use informatics.** Apply informatics to reducing errors, managing knowledge and information, decision-making, and communication.

Health Professions Education outlines some strategies to develop these competencies. Chapter 4 discusses each competency and the issues and information that should be considered per competency. This report influenced the funding for and the development of Quality and Safety in Nursing Education (QSEN).

A Summary of the February 2010 Forum on the Future of Nursing Education (2010)

This report focuses on nursing education and was incorporated into *The Future of Nursing*. Forums were held in several locations to get input from the nursing community, mostly from nursing faculty. The key topics were: what to teach, how to teach, and where to teach. Examples are provided in the content. Testimony from a variety of nursing leaders and other professionals is also provided. This report provides background for the information on nursing education included in *The Future of Nursing*. Some of the topics and suggestions are increased collaboration and communication with other health professions; use of systems thinking; care of the older adult in acute care and in the community; integration of technology such as simulation to develop problem-solving and critical thinking; and diversity across the lifespan. Nurse educators need to keep up-to-date with changes in health care delivery, partner with others in the community to improve student learning options and develop effective articulation agreements, and assist students in continuing their education to meet career goals as professionals. Not only was this content considered in *The Future of Nursing* report, but in reviewing *Educating Nurses: A Call for Radical Transformation* (Benner et al. 2010) one can also see similar themes.

Redesigning Continuing Education in the Health Professions (2010)

It is not surprising that, after addressing the issue of health care profession education from the perspective of degree programs, the attention would turn to the issue of lifelong learning for health care professionals. It is also significant that, just as with *Healthcare Professions Education*, the report addresses all health care professions in one report. Continuing education is used to ensure that health care professionals are up-to-date and can provide quality care based on current evidence. The report describes the key concern about the CE system: "As it is structured today, [CE] is so deeply flawed that it cannot properly support the development of health professionals. CE has become structured around health professional participation instead of performance improvement. This has left health professionals unprepared to consistently perform at the highest levels, putting into question whether the public is receiving care of the highest possible quality and safety" (IOM 2010a, ix). If CE is used effectively, the health care workforce can be strengthened and retooled, something that is critical to improving the quality of care. This report discusses the need for effective CE, the scientific foundations of CE, regulations and financing, and design and implementation of a new CE approach. The report provides useful information about current and possible future approaches to providing CE. This is of particular interest to those who are actively involved in continuing education programs. Another important topic is the evaluation of CE, something that has long been difficult do effectively. There is extensive discussion about the issue of licensure and CE requirements, which are not consistent either within each health care profession or across professions. Accreditation of CE programs is also described, and the report recognizes the need for consistent accreditation standards across professions and states.

Several options for designing a new model for CE are discussed; however, the report recommends that a public-private institute for CE professional development (CPD) be created. This recommendation has been made to the secretary of the HHS. Consideration should be given to content, regulation, financing, and the development and strengthening of a scientific basis for the practice of CPD. The CPD system should be based on the recommended five core competencies. To accomplish this will require greater interprofessional collaboration: "Imagine a healthcare system with the ability to rapidly adapt to the needs of patients, health professionals, and institutions through a shared commitment to CPD and high quality patient care.... Everyone is a learner, supported on the arc of professional development with knowledge of tailored learning goals, the tools to meet and surpass those goals, and a community of other learners with whom to share the process" (IOM 2010a, 111).

Building Health Workforce Capacity through Community-Based Health Professional Education: Workshop Summary (2014)

The purpose of this workshop was to encourage participants to consider different views of community so that this could be used to develop new approaches to teaching students (Cuff 2014b). This is important at a time when more emphasis is placed on public and community health and also the need for expanding prevention and health promotion activities across the life span. Emphasis is placed on getting students out into the community, away from structured settings such as clinics. The report includes a discussion about competencies. There is need to expand or spread innovations in community-based health professional learning across the continuum of education to practice. Additional discussion in this report focuses on outcomes and their impact.

Assessing Health Professional Education: Workshop Summary (2014)

Key terms that are used in this workshop and its report are *assessment* and *evaluation*. "Assessment is done to determine the level of understanding by a learner, while evaluation is a tool to determine how well a program or an educator teaching a course is conveying messages" (Cuff 2014a, 44). Consideration in assessment must be given to how learners learn and short- and long-term impact of the experience on knowledge and practice. The report covers a number of areas related to health professions education, including topics related to how best to integrate teamwork in education, such as simulation experiences. Other content focuses on the assessment of collaborative and transformational leadership; limitations in organizational cultures that inhibit collaboration; strategies for assessment; improving faculty development to support interprofessional practice and education; and strategies that might be used to engage faculty in interprofessional practice. Use of technology to engage patients and students is also discussed. Education assessment is reviewed from the perspectives of the macrolevel (policy), mesolevel (institution), and microlevel (individual).

Envisioning the Future of Health Professional Education: Workshop Summary (2016)

This report focuses on building a health workforce, redesigning and restructuring the curriculum, adjusting to a changing health workforce, and building a global health workforce (Cuff 2016). Health care education needs effective ways to cope with changing health care needs, practices, and technology. Interprofessional education (IPE) has an impact on health care profession education and offers challenges that require changes. There is concern that we are preparing students incorrectly and also wasting money in how we are doing it. Education needs to be more relevant. The report discusses each of these focus areas with examples.

Implications of the *Quality Chasm* Reports for Clinical Care

Taken together, the reports summarized in the first part of this book have many implications for clinical care and for health professions education in the United States. This final section examines the success of two ongoing, clinically-oriented initiatives that have been influenced by and reflect the recommendations from many of these reports: Transforming Care at the

Bedside (TCAB) initiative and the National Database of Nursing Quality Indicators (NDNQI) program. Other examples of programs and initiatives related to nursing and the *Quality Chasm* reports are the Magnet Recognition Program®, Nurses and HIT, 2016 Culture of Safety: It Starts with You, and the Nurses' Bill of Rights. We have to ask ourselves if we have improved care.

Transforming Care at the Bedside

Improving health care quality requires active participation from nurses—we provide care 24/7. The push to improve the quality of care comes at a critical time for nursing, and we have great need to make major improvements in nursing education. We need to be innovative. There is more to nursing than just filling positions. What can be done to transform care and make nursing more effective and efficient? We are witnessing a major technological explosion in health care, and we should make it work for us. The *Quality Chasm* reports have shown us that we—all health care professionals—need to work as teams. We need to recognize the value of the evidence we use to support our care decisions. We need more nursing research to solve real clinical problems. We need more QI initiatives that include active nursing participation. Some priority setting is also required so that our efforts will be efficient and effective.

The TCAB initiative began formally in 2003 with funding and support from the Robert Wood Johnson Foundation (RWJF) and the Institute for Healthcare Improvement (IHI) (IHI 2008e, 2011). This is a collaborative effort to redesign the work environment of nurses and to involve nurses directly in that transformation. TCAB relates to *Keeping Patients Safe* and *The Future of Nursing* report. It uses a QI approach that engages frontline staff and unit managers working as teams. In this initiative, staff and unit managers drive problem identification for improvement. Medical-surgical units in acute care were chosen as the settings for the first pilots in the initiative, with three hospitals included in the initial phase, and now many more are running pilots. TCAB is based on four main components (IHI 2011): safe and reliable care, vitality and teamwork, patient-centered care, and value-added care processes.

Embedded within TCAB is the language of the *Quality Chasm* series, including the overall goal of care improvement and quality care. The initiative includes the following "tests of change" (Martin et al. 2007, 445):

- Redesign the work environment, focusing on the staff who do the work and where they do the work.
- Create improvement focused on the needs of patients and staff.

- Provide support from executive leadership.
- Test first with a small sample, learn, and then extend use to other areas.
- Understand that this is an opportunity for learning.

A key drive is to make effective change happen as soon as possible.

The TCAB process uses deep dive or total immersion into a problem to explore, brainstorm, and prioritize. Staff members are asked this question: "If you could create the perfect patient and staff experience, what would it look like? Consider the key design themes in guiding your thoughts and ideas. If you find yourself focusing on current problems, push your mind to think of a solution or another way to design it" (Martin et al. 2007, 445). Apply this to the following six-step process (445):

1. Describe the current state of the problem; include key stakeholders' views.
2. Examine the root problem to increasing understanding.
3. Select a process to focus on.
4. Identify intervention(s) to use, such as Plan, Do, Check, Act (PDCA).
5. Begin small and rapidly move and test, identifying what is not working and adapting as you go along.
6. Determine best approach(es) to improvements, then apply them to larger areas (more units, organization-wide, and so on).

During the TCAB process, staff may identify some changes that need to be done immediately, referred to as "just-do-its." These should be applied when identified. The TCAB framework can be found at the IHI website (IHI 2017b).

Nursing Data on Quality Care: NDNQI

In 1994, the American Nurses Association (ANA) began an investigation of the impact of workforce restructuring and redesign on the safety and quality of patient care in acute care settings. ANA wanted to "explore the nature and strength of the linkages between nursing care and patient outcomes by identifying nursing quality indicators" (Pollard, Mitra, and Mendelson 1996, 1). A system was designed to educate nurses, consumers, and policymakers about nursing's contributions in the acute care setting, focusing on monitoring the quality of nursing care. Patients come into the acute care setting primarily because they need 24/7 care, which is the focus of nursing. This early study made it clear that there was a lack of data about nursing, outcomes, and nursing-sensitive indicators. Old methods of collecting data were not nursing specific. This project identified ten "nursing-sensitive indicators" that reflected characteristics of the nursing workforce, nursing processes, or patient outcomes.

After the 1994 survey, ANA, in collaboration with seven state nurses' associations, conducted a pilot to determine whether it was possible to collect data on the indicators from a large number of sites. In 1998, after this pilot, the ANA established the NDNQI.

Today, more than 1,500 hospitals participate in this database, providing "each nurse the opportunity to review the evidence, evaluate their practice, and determine what improvements can be made" (Montalvo and Dunton 2007, 3). More than 300,000 nurses provide data based on these indicators, staffing data, and RN survey data focused on the unit-level of care. The participating hospitals submit their nursing-sensitive indicator data to the NDNQI database. The NDNQI's nursing-sensitive indicators focus on structure, process, and outcomes. Press Ganey now manages the database (http://www.pressganey.com/solutions/clinical-quality/nursing-quality).

The data are available for research and analysis of nursing-specific quality services. The Centers of Medicare and Medicaid Services (CMS) requires hospitals to participate in a systematic clinical database registry for nursing-sensitive care. Some states require this monitoring, though it is not yet required nationally. Magnet Recognition hospitals must participate in the NDNQI database process.

Taxonomy of Error, Root Cause Analysis, and Practice Responsibility (TERCAP)

The National Council for State Boards of Nursing (NCSBN) developed a database to increase understanding and availability of data on nursing errors, the Taxonomy of Error, Root Cause Analysis, and Practice Responsibility (TERCAP®) (NCSBN 2016b). It is an error reporting system and different from the NDNQI, which is based on indicators and results. It is a voluntary system, and not all states participate. The practice areas focused on in the database are medication administration, communicating patient data, attentiveness and surveillance, clinical reasoning and judgment, prevention, intervention, interpretation of orders, and professional responsibility. The TERCAP website provides details and current information about this important error tracking program, the only one for nursing errors (NCSBN 2016b). This database relates directly back to the *Quality Chasm* reports as it is based on the five health care professions core competencies and the later work done by QSEN.

ANA Position Statements and Guides for Safety for Nurses

The ANA provides a number of resources that are related to the work described in this part of the book. The ANA website provides information and position statements focused on a healthy work environment: "A Healthy Work Environment is one that is safe, empowering, and satisfying. Parallel to the World Health Organization definition of health, it is not merely the absence of real and perceived threats to health, but a place of physical, mental, and social well-being, supporting optimal health and safety" (ANA 2016c). Examples of some of the topics covered on the website are nurse fatigue, handling of drugs, and bullying and workplace violence.

The second topic that is connected to this content is called Healthy Nurse, Healthy Nation™. Healthy nurses are better able to provide quality care and maintain safety for patients and themselves. The ANA website provides more information and updates on this topic (ANA 2016b).

Magnet Recognition Program

The Magnet Recognition Program was initiated in the early 1980s and has been influenced by the *Quality Chasm* reports, core competencies and QSEN competencies, initiatives from HHS, the Triple Aim and STEEEP, and the importance of structure, process, and outcomes, as well as others. This program awards the highest organizational credential for nursing excellence (Robert and Finlayson 2015). The ANCC administrates this program and its website provides information about the process (http://www.nursecredentialing.org/Magnet). Figure 1-1 describes the Magnet model. The model focuses on the 14 Forces of Magnetism, identified in table 1-1. Students should be familiar with this program and understand how it relates to quality care and roles of nurses. They should consider the Forces of Magnetism as criteria of excellence that can help them when they decide on employment—how do potential employers demonstrate the forces even if they are not a Magnet HCO? The ANCC provides a number of resources about important information related to the major criteria for this recognition (ANCC 2013a, 2013b, 2013c, 2013d, 2013e). The process to reach Magnet status is long and requires much work on the part of nurses and nursing leadership within the HCO. HCOs must demonstrate excellent nursing processes, quality patient care, and a high level of patient satisfaction, and must strive to improve the education level of its nurses.

Nurses and HIT

Nurses are more and more involved in HIT, as providers who use HIT, as providers who are involved in quality improvement initiatives that require use of HIT and data, and as informatics nurses, a nursing specialty. The specialty role is relatively new. In 2015 the Healthcare Information and Management Systems Society (HIMSS) conducted a survey that was a follow-up to its 2009 survey of informatics nurses (HIMSS 2015). The survey included responses from 576 nurses who responded to questions related to quality of patient care, direct impact on clinical systems, hiring informatics professionals, executive leadership, longevity, and involvement of informatics nurses in emerging technologies. The results indicate that these nurses feel their greatest value is in the implementation phase and optimization phase of the clinical systems process. Nurses, and nurses with special training, do offer a lot to HIT. Having a basic understanding of HIT and its relevance is important for all nurses.

We are also influenced by federal initiatives that should guide policy and practice. An example is the *Federal Health IT Strategic Plan 2015-2020* (ONC 2015). The plan includes four overarching goals that are interdependent: (1) Advance person-centered and self-managed health, (2) transform health care delivery and community health, (3) foster research, scientific knowledge, and innovation, and (4) enhance the nation's HIT infrastructure. The vision is "high-quality care, lower costs, healthy population, and engaged people," and the mission is to "improve the health and well-being of individuals and communities through the use of technology and health

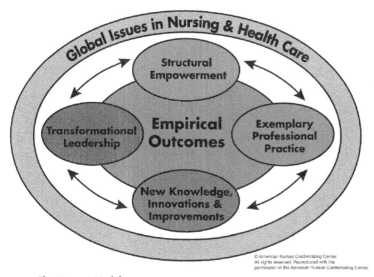

FIGURE 1-1. **The Magnet Model.**
    Source: American Nurses Credentialing Center. 2013. *Empirical Outcomes: Criteria for Nursing Excellence.* Silver Spring, MD: American Nurses Credentialing Center.

Table 1.1   Forces of Magnetism and Derivation of The Magnet Model

Forces of Magnetism	Empirical Domains of Evidence	Magnet Model Components
1. Quality of Nursing Leadership 3. Management Style	Leadership	Transformational Leadership
2. Organizational Structure 4. Personnel Policies and Programs 10. Community and Health Care Organization 12. Image of Nursing 14. Professional Development	Resource Utilization and Development	Structural Empowerment
5. Professional Models of Care 8. Consultation and Resources 9. Autonomy 11. Nurses as Teachers 13. Interdisciplinary (Interprofessional) Relationships 6. Quality of Care: Ethics, Patient Safety, and Quality Infrastructure 7. Quality Improvement	Professional Practice Model Safe and Ethical Practice Autonomous Practice Quality Processes	Exemplary Professional Practice
6. Quality of Care: Research- and Evidence-Based Practice 7. Quality Improvement	Research	Knew Knowledge, Innovations & Improvements
6. Quality of Care	Outcomes	Empirical Quality Outcomes

Source: American Nurses Credentialing Center. 2013. *Empirical Outcomes: Criteria for Nursing Excellence.* Silver Spring, MD: American Nurses Credentialing Center.

information that is accessible when and where it matters most" (ONC 2015). The vision described integrates STEEEP. HealthIT.gov provides updates on this work and resources that can be used to prepare nurses for HIT.

2016 Culture of Safety: It Starts with You

ANA chose a significant theme for 2016: "Culture of Safety: It Starts with You" (ANA 2016a). This decision recognizes the importance of quality care including the element of safety in health care delivery and relevance to nurses as key health care staff. It also focuses on the responsibility of each nurse and the profession. ANA bases this decision on the results of *Quality Chasm* series and the need to improve care. Its website provides additional information on this initiative, with each month focusing on different topics related to the theme.

Nurses' Bill of Rights

ANA developed a bill of rights for nurses. This is associated with a healthy workplace and recognizes the important role of nurses. To accomplish this nurses must be supported and know what their rights are as professionals. The ANA Bill of Rights for registered Nurses reads as follows (ANA 2016f):

> *To maximize the contributions nurses make to society, it is necessary to protect the dignity and autonomy of nurses in the workplace. To that end, the following rights must be afforded:*

> 1. *Nurses have the right to practice in a manner that fulfills their obligations to society and to those who receive nursing care.*
> 2. *Nurses have the right to practice in environments that allow them to act in accordance with professional standards and legally authorized scopes of practice.*
> 3. *Nurses have the right to a work environment that supports and facilitates ethical practice, in accordance with the Code of Ethics for Nurses with Interpretive Statements.*
> 4. *Nurses have the right to freely and openly advocate for themselves and their patients, without fear of retribution.*
> 5. *Nurses have the right to fair compensation for their work, consistent with their knowledge, experience, and professional responsibilities.*
> 6. *Nurses have the right to a work environment that is safe for themselves and for their patients.*
> 7. *Nurses have the right to negotiate the conditions of their employment, either as individuals or collectively, in all practice settings.*

Have We Improved Health Care?

One has to ask whether health care in the United States has improved since the publication of the first edition of this book in 2007 and throughout subsequent editions—or even since publication of the first *Quality Chasm* report in 1999. The CMS, as a key health care agency in the HHS, notes:

We all know what we want our healthcare system to deliver: the right care for every patient every time. As the Institute of Medicine has defined it, high-quality care is care that is safe, effective, efficient, patient-centered, timely, and equitable. And with continuing medical progress, the potential for care that is even better in all of these dimensions is increasingly possible.

Increasingly, we are finding that high quality means care that is personalized, prevention-oriented, and patient-centered, based on evidence about the benefits and costs for each particular patient. This is the direction of twenty-first century biomedical science, science that is marked by new approaches in the lab like genomics, or nanotechnology, or next-generation information technology and more personalized medicine. These new sciences are only just beginning to have an impact on patient care, but they hold tremendous potential.

We also know that there are large gaps, even a chasm, between our goal of high-quality care for every patient every time and what our healthcare system delivers. We have the potential for the best health care in the world—and in so many ways we achieve it, every day, thanks to the talent and commitment and hard work of health professionals, and researchers and product developers, and so many people who work every day to improve the health of Americans. But too often and in too many ways, these dedicated people—who amount to the world's greatest asset for improving public health—are frustrated in their efforts to achieve the goal of closing the gap. (CMS 2007)

The *Quality Chasm* series makes the point that we have many areas of concern in health care delivery, such as patient-centered care; effective, efficient, timely care; quality improvement and the need for evidence; HIT; diversity and disparity; and more. The first quality report was published in 1999, but problems continue today. We have much more work to do.

Other data also indicate that the United States continues to have major quality care problems. Harvey Fineberg, a past president of the HMD who was very instrumental in the development of the *Quality Chasm* series, has the following to say about a successful health system, emphasizing the critical elements for the series: the system has "three attributes: healthy people, meaning a population that attains the highest level of health possible; superior care, meaning care that is effective, safe, timely, patient-centered, equitable, and efficient; and fairness, meaning that treatment is applied without discrimination or disparities to all individuals and families, regardless of age, group identity, or place, and that the system is fair to the health professions, institutions, and businesses supporting and delivering care" (Fineberg 2012, 1020).

We do know that health care quality has improved, but more improvement is needed. For example, between 2010 and 2013 there were 17 percent fewer harms to patients and an estimated fewer hospital-acquired conditions (Kronick 2015). The World Health Organization (WHO) provides current data about global health, including the United States. The data are useful in comparing countries, for example, life expectancy reported for the United States is 79.3 years. Many other countries are doing much better. In the Americas, Canada (82.2) and Chile (80.5) beat life expectancy in the United States. There are twenty-one European countries with longer life expectancies than the United States, ranging from Cyprus (80.5) to Switzerland (83.4). In the Western Pacific Region there are five countries where life expectancies are greater than in the United States: Japan (topping the charts at 83.7), Singapore (83.1), Australia (82.8), Republic of Korea (82.3), and New Zealand (81.6; WHO 2016b, 8).

Summing Up: *Quality Chasm* and Other IOM/HMD Reports

The major reports from the *Quality Chasm* series provide important data and recommendations that will help to improve health care quality and safety nationally, if applied. The reports begin with a critical examination of health care safety and quality, and proceed to

- Develop frameworks and terminology for data analysis, action plans, and reporting mechanisms;
- Define the role of leadership, particularly the role of government;
- Explore critical issues related to public and community health and diversity;
- Specify the priorities of quality improvement initiatives;
- Monitor health care quality and disparities;
- Analyze the nursing workplace; and
- Examine health professions education and identify core competencies for all health professions.

As this chapter indicates, there have been many more reports published since the first *Quality Chasm* reports expanding on the examination of quality from multiple perspectives. Though published separately, the reports do not stand alone; rather, each expands on previous reports in the quality care series. Key terminology (definitions for quality and safety, application of STEEP, and so on) is consistent from one report to the next. This interconnectedness makes it important to understand the general information in each report, how the reports relate, and the recommendations and their implications for nursing and health care. Figure 1-2 provides an overview of the development of the initial critical reports in the *Quality Chasm* reports.

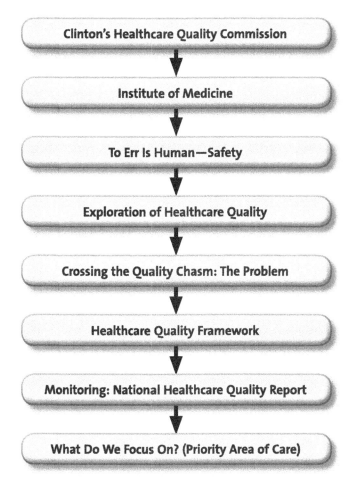

FIGURE 1-2. Development of the *Quality Chasm* series

2

Implications of Health Care Reform for Nursing Education

Chapter 1 discussed the many reports and initiatives from the National Academies of Sciences, Engineering, and Medicine (the National Academies) Health and Medicine Division (HMD), formerly known as the Institute of Medicine (IOM), and their impact on health care policy, delivery of care, and health care professions. The earlier reports, beginning in 1999, clearly set the stage for later policy development and influenced some of the provisions in the Patient Protection and Affordable Care Act of 2010, known as the ACA. Chapter 2 follows this story into the Obama administration's work to implement health care reform, the uncertain fate of the ACA following the 2016 election, the role and responsibilities of the US Department of Health and Human Services (HHS), and the development of an important national initiative, the National Quality Strategy (NQS).

The Obama Administration and the Affordable Care Act

Not too long after the election of President Obama in 2008 and the beginning of his administration in 2009, one heard the term "perfect storm" applied to the next phase of US health care. This phrase implies a perspective that could have serious negative consequences, along with the potential opportunity for significant and comprehensive reform that has not been available for many years. In 2009, there was an intense nationwide expectation of change that closely matched the need for such change. The Obama administration's initial response was to identify key health care principles that would guide its health care reform decision-making (Politico 2009):

- Protect families' financial health
- Make health coverage affordable
- Aim for universality
- Provide portability of coverage
- Guarantee choice
- Invest in prevention and wellness
- Improve patient safety and quality of care
- Maintain long-term fiscal sustainability

There is no doubt the United States has been in an ongoing health care crisis for some time. In 2008, Enthoven noted that health care costs were draining the budget, and he believed it would take a major health care organization (HCO) change to control this cost (Enthoven 2008). In 2014, health care costs increased by 5.3 percent compared to 2013—with total of $3 trillion overall. Federal government health care costs alone rose by 11.7 percent to nearly $844 billion, as noted by the HHS (Pianin 2015). This time period follows the initial implementation of the ACA. The *Quality Chasm* reports and subsequent reports provide even greater evidence of the need for change.

- The *Quality Chasm* series describes a dysfunctional, fragmented health care system that is not yielding positive outcomes, either in cost or in quality.
- A growing number of citizens do not have health care coverage, and others have inadequate coverage.
- An increasing number of people must deal with chronic illnesses and the complex care needs.

- There is fluctuating shortage of health care providers (nurses and others), which can occur in a geographic location or in a specific HCO and will increase as more providers retire.
- There is greater integration of quality improvement (QI) preparation for all health care professions.
- The aging population requires more health care services, and this need will increase.
- The cost of care is still rising rapidly—for the government, for employers, and for individuals.
- There continue to be serious disparities in the delivery and outcomes of health care.
- Health promotion and prevention need to be expanded across all populations.

Even though we have much knowledge and many tools (e.g, drugs, treatment, technology, and so on) to ensure that we provide quality, we are not successful enough. In some cases these opportunities have increased the cost of care. This list was prepared for the first edition of this book, and it is still relevant for the fourth edition, though revised some.

President Obama's move for health care reform was hardly the first. Tom Daschle, a US senator for many years, and coauthors provided an overview of the very long history of US attempts and failures to reform health care—going back to the development of health care reimbursement in the early twentieth century to later increased federal government roles through Medicare and Medicaid (Daschle, Lambrew, and Greenberger 2008). His description remains useful to better understand the historical perspective of health care issues. As Daschle notes, we have not been successful: "Our system is fundamentally broken, and decades of failed incremental measures have proven that we need a comprehensive approach to fix it" (xiv). He even describes the efforts as the "tortuous history of health reform" (45). Why have we not succeeded in improving the system? Daschle believes the traditional legislative process cannot deliver the changes we need. It has failed many times to do so even when the broad framework of a plan is acceptable. The ideal framework is described as "a public-private hybrid that preserves our private system within a strengthened public framework" (107).

In 2010, the Patient Protection and Affordable Care Act (Pub. L. No. 11-148) and the Health Care and Education Reconciliation Act (Pub. L. No. 111-152) were passed, initiating the current movement in health care reform. This legislation came to be commonly referred to as the Affordable

Care Act or the ACA, ObamaCare by some. In June 2012 and also in another later case, the US Supreme Court upheld the constitutionality of most of the law's provisions. There continued to be issues with the effort to increase insurance coverage, although universal health care coverage was not part of this effort. At the time of the publication of this book, this law was under review by the Trump administration and Congress. It is, however, important for nurses understand the ACA, what it is and its impact, even if major changes are made or it is eliminated. The following offers a review of recent developments in the law and their impact.

In 2016 and continuing in 2017, several of the major insurers had pulled out of the plan options under the ACA for a variety of reasons. The impact of these changes is serious; however, some insurers claim they are losing money due to the impact of too many members who have health problems since those who are healthier, particularly younger adults, are not signing up for the plans and are choosing to pay the penalty fee. When the ACA was developed there was a concern that this would happen. Premiums have increased and are expected to increase more in 2017. In 2016, there were half as many people in the insurance exchanges as had been predicted (Abelson and Sanger-Katz 2016).

Due to the changing nature of the topic of health care reimbursement, the ACA, and what might be done in the future, this is a topic that requires nurses to keep up-to-date with health policy changes due to potential future changes and, when possible, to participate actively in further policy development. It is a topic that is also very political.

We tend to focus on the reimbursement aspects of the ACA; however, we should not forget its other provisions, which may be lost if the law is eliminated or changed. When one reads the ACA, it is easy to see the influence of the *Quality Chasm* reports on health care legislation. Although the law is primarily about health care reimbursement and providing coverage for more people (though not universal health care coverage), it does include other provisions. Nurses need to know about the provisions and their implications for nursing. The laws support nursing in many ways: providing funding for workforce development, developing nurse-managed clinics, using more home-care services, developing and implementing QI strategies, emphasizing community-based collaboration and higher quality, accessible mental health care, implementing wellness and preventive services, emphasizing health promotion and primary care, and more. Increasing access to care also has direct implications for nursing, such as the increasing need for more nurses and changes in the settings where nurses may work.

Examples of provisions that are QI oriented are listed below:

- The mandated development of the National Quality Strategy (NQS), with annual status reports to be given to Congress. These reports must also reflect the results of the annual National Healthcare Quality and Disparities Report (QDR);
- Greater focus on comparative effectiveness research; establishing the Patient-Centered Outcomes Research (PCORI);
- Greater emphasis on care coordination for Medicare and Medicaid patients;
- Establishment of a National Workforce Commission (this effort has not been very effective since the law was passed with limited funding allocated);
- Establishment of more effective data collection related to health care disparities;
- Development and improvement of national uniform standards for health plans and electronic exchange of health information;
- Increased emphasis on prevention and health promotion through the development of programs that support greater coverage for them in health plans; and
- Development of community-based transition programs.

The ACA also supports greater use of electronic medical or health records (EMRs/EHRs) in all health care settings, emphasizing the importance of health informatics technology (HIT). We need more funding, research and demonstration projects, and monitoring of health care outcomes to develop effective use of HIT. HIT has expanded rapidly since 2010, and the HHS is very active in developing and managing initiatives to improve HIT and increase its use by HCOs and other health care providers.

In 2016, a number of reviews of the current status of the ACA were published in the *Journal of the American Medical Association*, including an opinion piece by President Obama discussing his administration's current perspective of the effects of the ACA based on data (Obama 2016, 525):

- There has been an increase in insurance coverage; the uninsured rate decreased from 16 percent in 2010 to 9.1 percent in 2015, a relative decrease of 43 percent.
- States that expanded their Medicaid programs as part of the ACA decreased their uninsured rates from 2013 to 2015, with a greater impact on states with a history of greater numbers of uninsured people.

- Early evidence suggests that expanded coverage has led to some improvement in access to treatment, financial security, and health.
- Payer spending per health care enrollee continues to decrease and health care quality has improved.

What will happen with these important provisions? The new administration has already made changes that impact QI; for example, the Agency for Healthcare Research and Quality, has been moved from the HHS to the National Institutes of Health. The AHRQ is a critical source for efforts to improve care, and even more so following the passage of the ACA. A critical question that arises from this: Will AHRQ lose funding? What would this do to its proven track record as a strong resource supporting the development of QI? This serves as a good example of what can happen with changes that are not directly or even indirectly related to health care reimbursement. Nurses must monitor changes and also speak up providing leadership to ensure we are moving forward in providing the best quality care and the most reasonable cost. We cannot now predict what will happen with the ACA nor is it appropriate to focus in this book on proposed changes that are only in discussion and not fully approved. This responsibility lies with faculty, students, and nurses to keep up-to-date on this topic. Some resources for this are listed in the text box on the next page, "Health Care Reform and Policy: Some Online Resources."

US Department of Health and Human Services Reforms

As was mentioned, a number of issues and initiatives have been coming together at the same time. As is true for some of the other *Quality Chasm* reports, *HHS in the 21st Century: Charting a New Course for a Healthier America* was initiated in response to a congressional request, in this case on June 20, 2007, from the Congressional Committee on Oversight and Government Reform (Schaeffer, Schultz, and Salerno 2009). The committee's request included several key questions aimed at providing a better understanding of some of the concerns about the HHS (162):

- What are the missions of the HHS and its individual agencies, and how do these missions relate to the challenges confronting us?
- How effectively are the HHS agencies organized to achieve their mission?
- Could the missions of individual HHS agencies be consolidated or realigned to make them more effective?
- What recommendations would the HMD make to Congress and the HHS to improve the focus of individual agencies, enhance their accountability, and improve their efficiency?

Health Care Reform and Policy: Some Online Resources

Agency for Healthcare Research and Quality
(https://www.ahrq.gov/news/index.html)

A newsletter, blog, news releases, and social media options available from this page supplement AHRQ's reports and other resources on such health care delivery topics as access to care and health care utilization (https://www.ahrq.gov/topics/index.html)

American Nurses Association (http://www.nursingworld.org/ MainMenuCategories/Policy-Advocacy/HealthSystemReform)

This is one of several ANA offerings of information on health policy and advocacy issues from the perspective and for the benefit of registered nurses. ANA's "Principles for Health System Transformation 2016" frames content on both current and past topics.

Centers for Medicare and Medicaid Services (https://www.cms.gov/ Outreach-and-Education/Outreach-and-Education.html)

This page allows quick access to health policy topics, the "ACA and Marketplace" being foremost in this context. The CMS newsroom can be accessed from this page as well.

Families USA (http://familiesusa.org/)

An avowed advocacy organization that calls itself "the voice of health-care consumers," their site offers extensive resources for the interested and activist citizen; its Resource Library features a useful filter to quickly locate specific information. A worthy supplement to Kaiser Health News.

Kaiser Health News (http://khn.org/)

A robust source of in-depth information on and insight into health care policy and politics and workings the health care system. Their daily KHN Morning Briefing on the opening page is a good place to start.

National League for Nursing (http://www.nln.org/advocacy-public-policy)

The NLN represents nurse faculty and other leaders in nursing education. Their policy and advocacy resources focus on shaping and influencing policies that affect nursing workforce development. Under "Legislative Issues," the "Access" and "Workforce" links are most pertinent to the topics in chapter 2.

- What recommendations would the HMD make to more effectively integrate the promotion of public health and control of health care costs across the department?

The committee of experts that examined the HHS did not recommend a major reorganization of the HHS, but rather described an approach to transform the department focusing on five key areas (Schaeffer, Schultz, and Salerno 2009).

1. Define a twenty-first-century vision.
2. Foster adaptability and alignment.
3. Increase the effectiveness and efficiency of the US health care system.
4. Strengthen the HHS and US public health and health care workforces.
5. Improve accountability and decision-making.

Why should nurses care about a report that examines the HHS? First, it is important to recognize that the HHS is the largest federal government agency, based on budget. The department has an impact on every American. Its activities are extremely broad and conducted through the work of its multiple agencies, which is also one of its problems. Through this department flow decisions related to HHS resources: the Health Resources and Services Administration (HRSA), for example, focuses on health care education, funding (such as grants for research), and funding for the National Institutes of Health (NIH); the Agency for Healthcare Research and Quality (AHRQ) focuses on health care quality; the Food and Drug Administration (FDA) focuses on food and drug safety including some aspects of medical technology; the Indian Health Service (IHS) focuses on providing health care services to Native American populations; the Substance Abuse and Mental Health Services Administration (SAMHSA) focuses on research and services for these health needs; the Centers for Disease Control and Prevention (CDC) emphasizes data and monitoring, epidemiology, and QI; and the highly important Centers for Medicare and Medicaid Services (CMS) focus on administration and reimbursement of services for Medicare and Medicaid populations. Just reviewing these agencies within the department indicates the impact the HHS has on the entire nation, and all are involved in some aspects of quality improvement. Nursing is involved in all of the areas governed by these agencies, which affects our education, practice, and research. We need to be more involved in changes that might be made in the HHS and its functions.

The scope of HHS responsibilities and challenges is very large and significant. The recommendations from the report on the HHS are connected to issues raised in previous reports in the *Quality Chasm* series: more research and quality, evidence-based practice; patient-centered care; health care informatics; workforce issues; an integrative public health agenda; diversity and disparity; aging population; increase in chronic illness; the impact of quality improvement; the need for health promotion and prevention; and more. The HHS needs to focus on current and future needs that have become clearer since the publication of *To Err Is Human* (Kohn, Corrigan, and Donaldson 1999).

The current strategic plan for HHS is for 2014–18. The plan is available on the HHS website (HHS 2015), where it is updated periodically. The goals are to

1. Strengthen health care,
2. Advance scientific knowledge and innovation,
3. Advance the health, safety, and well-being of the American people, and
4. Ensure efficiency, transparency, and accountability of HHS programs.

The HHS mission is "to enhance the health and well-being of Americans by providing effective health and human services and by fostering sound, sustained advances in the sciences underlying medicine, public health and social services" (HHS 2015). The HHS is often charged with developing regulations for legislation and implementing health care–related legislation; for example:

- The American Recovery and Reinvestment Act of 2009 (ARRA) includes provisions on health care costs, payments, and HIT; ensures that programs awarded funding meet the law's requirements; measures program performance and ensures program integrity; and informs the public of results.
- The ACA includes, for example, the provisions noted in this chapter on pages 68–71.

Laws like these guide the work of the HHS and its organization, function, and priorities.

The National Quality Strategy

The ACA includes a provision to develop and implement a national health care quality framework (Burstin, Leatherman, and Goldmann 2016). The HHS assigned the AHRQ to take on these tasks. The AHRQ used the

Triple Aim, incorporating STEEEP (safety, timely, effectiveness, efficiency, equality, and patient-centeredness) to develop the NQS framework. The Triple Aim includes (AHRQ 2017a):

1. **Better Care:** Improve the overall quality by making health care more patient-centered, reliable, accessible, and safe.
2. **Healthy People / Healthy Communities:** Improve the health of the US population by supporting proven interventions to address behavioral, social, and environmental determinants of health in addition to delivering higher-quality care.
3. **Affordable Care:** Reduce the cost of quality health care for individuals, families, employers, and government.

Figure 2-1 provides an overview of the NQS. This framework is used along with the QDR to monitor care and an annual status report to Congress is required. It is suggested that the health care delivery system adopt and implement the NQS (framework and tools). This cannot be required, but is recommended. Nursing also needs to integrate this framework and the NQS tools. We need to consider how the NQS applies to nursing education, practice, and research. The *Quality Chasm* series influences the NQS as a driver in getting to the point of developing this framework and integrating the message that QI is critical in health care delivery.

Chapter 2 content expands on content in chapter 1 by emphasizing changes due to health care reform and other aspects of national health care policy, all of which are important to the nursing profession. Chapter 3 will focus on the importance of the nursing profession, its standards, and other relevant statements that guide nursing practice. All of these are connected to the critical issues found in chapters 1 and 2.

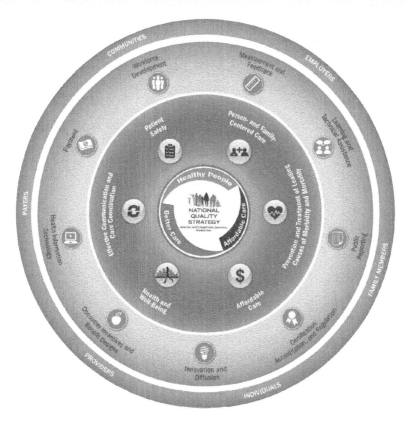

FIGURE 2-1. **National Quality Strategy: How It Works**
Source: Agency for Healthcare Research and Quality 2017b. National Quality Strategy Stakeholder Toolkit; p. 10.

3

Connecting the Reports to Nursing Standards and Ethics

As a profession, nursing has its own standards, code of ethics, and other policy and practice documents. There is a relationship between the Institute of Medicine (IOM) and the Health and Medicine Division's (HMD) ongoing efforts to improve care and the nursing profession's development of critical nursing statements about the profession and its roles in health care delivery. The following content provides an overview of this relationship in an effort to further explicate the connection between these important professional statements and the need to improve the health care system and the quality of care. As will be noted in more detail in later chapters of this book, the HMD strongly supports the integration of its five core competencies for the health care professions into all health care education. (See the discussion in chapter 1 of the 2003 IOM report *Health Professions Education*, the source of these core competencies.) Standards, which include professional and practice standards, are a part of quality improvement (QI), which is a continuous process (CQI).

Nursing's Social Policy Statement

The American Nurses Association's (ANA) social policy statement recognizes that nursing has an obligation to the public and the community. These social concerns influence how nurses practice and nurses' authority to practice. Social concerns in health care and nursing are related to the concerns discussed in many of the *Quality Chasm* series of reports. The 2010 ANA social policy statement is now published as an appendix in *Nursing: Scope and Standards of Practice*, 3rd edition (ANA 2015c, 180–84).

The following lists the social concerns of which the profession must be cognizant and on which nursing professionals must provide leadership. These areas are identified with their related health care profession core competencies:

- **Organization, delivery, and financing of quality health care** (relates to the core competencies of quality improvement, informatics, and evidence-based practice)
- **Provision for the public's health** (relates to the core competencies of patient-centered care and interprofessional teamwork)
- **Expansion of nursing and health care knowledge and appropriate application of technology** (relates to the core competencies of evidence-based practice and informatics)
- **Expansion of health care resources and health policy** (relates to the core competency of quality improvement)
- **Definitive planning for health care policy and regulation** (relates to the core competencies of patient-centered care, quality improvement, and interprofessional teamwork)
- **Duties under extreme conditions** (relates to the core competency of patient-centered care)

As a profession, we have a social responsibility and a social contract with our patients, whether they are individuals, families, or communities and populations. This contract implies two partners. Patient-centered care is central, and although this term is not used in the ANA social policy statement, it is implied. The other core competencies (quality improvement, interprofessional teamwork, informatics, and evidence-based practice) are all interwoven in the social context in which practice takes place and are required for professional nursing to be effective.

Professional collaboration is discussed in the social policy statement, which describes collaboration as "true partnership, valuing expertise, power, and respect on all sides and recognizing and accepting separate and combined spheres of activity and responsibility. Collaboration includes mutual safeguarding of the legitimate interests of each party and commonality of goals that is recognized by all parties" (ANA 2015c, 185). Faculty need to do more to prepare students for this type of collaboration; they also need to model this type of collaboration for students. We must emphasize the positive in other health care professions. Rather than sharing our negative stories of how we are victims—we are not asked for our advice, we are not viewed as members of the professional team, and so on—we need to tell stories of effective collaboration and how to make it better. Our social contract says we must do this as a profession.

Guide to Nursing's Social Policy Statement: Understanding the Profession from Social Contract to Social Covenant (Fowler 2015b) is a companion ANA document that expands on nurses' understanding of the nursing profession, both in terms of its social contract and the transformation of that contract into a social covenant. This guide not only discusses our roles as a profession, but also what we should expect from society and the government (local, state, national). This discussion describes sixteen elements of the social contract, which are reciprocal between nursing and society (Fowler 2015b, 19–22). They are included here (see page 80) so that they can be reviewed and considered in the context of their connections to the *Quality Chasm* reports, the five health care profession core competencies, and other initiatives to improve care for society, whether that be for individuals, families, local communities, states, the nation, or globally.

This guide discusses other issues related to the social contract that are important for students to consider as they enter the profession or as they advance their education and practice. Among these is civic professionalism, which "puts public service, the welfare of the public, and the professional–public partnership at the heart of the profession's involvement with society. It seeks to further social goods such as health, solidarity, equality, equity, and dignity" (Fowler 2015b, 70). To accomplish this we need nursing leadership based on professional standards and ethics, and engagement in the process of QI for patients, wherever they may be.

Nursing: Scope and Standards of Practice (2015)

The ANA professional nursing standards (ANA 2015c) go hand-in-hand with the social policy statement. The definition of nursing can also be connected to the *Quality Chasm* reports: "Nursing is the protection, promotion, and optimization of health and abilities, prevention of illness and injury, alleviation of suffering through the diagnosis and treatment of human response, and advocacy in the care of individuals, families,

The Elements of Nursing's Social Contract

Society's Expectations of Nursing within the Social Contract

1. Caring service
2. Primacy of the patient
3. Knowledge, skill, and competence
4. Hazardous service
5. Responsibility and accountability
6. Progress and development
7. Ethical practice
8. Collaboration
9. Promotion of health of the public

Nursing's Expectations of Society within the Social Contract

1. Autonomy of practice
2. Self-governance
3. Title and practice protection
4. Respect and just remuneration
5. Freedom to practice
6. Workforce sustainability
7. Protection in hazardous service

communities, and populations" (ANA 2015c, 1). To meet this definition, nurses must be competent.

Competency is "an expected level of performance that integrates knowledge, skills, abilities, and judgment" (ANA 2015c, 44). The health care profession core competencies are designed for all health care professions, including nursing. The competencies are the basic starting points and do not negate the need for competencies focused on specific professions such as nursing, medicine, and pharmacy. For example, there are the Quality and Safety Education for Nurses (QSEN) competencies. As we develop our curricula and courses, then, we must ensure that these five competencies are included. To meet the nursing profession standards, we must also meet these other competencies.

A necessary context for understanding nursing standards is the scope of nursing practice—the who, what, where, when, why, and how of nursing practice. State nurse practice acts also address these questions. Many nursing specialties also have specific standards for their practice areas. They are not discussed here but are important.

The nursing standards are based on tenets characteristic of nursing practice (ANA 2015c, 7):

1. Caring and health are central to the practice of the registered nurse.
2. Nursing practice is individualized.
3. Registered nurses use the nursing process to plan and provide individualized care for health care consumers.
4. Nurses coordinate care by establishing partnerships.
5. A strong link exists between the professional work environment and the registered nurse's ability to provide quality health care and achieve optimal outcomes.

All of these tenets can be connected to the need today for effective implementation of the nursing process, teamwork, quality improvement, and professional development to ensure practice competencies are met.

In its Model of Professional Nursing Practice Regulation (ANA 2015c), the ANA integrates key elements that are also found in the *Quality Chasm* reports and the five health care profession core competencies. We need quality care that is safe for both the patient and the employee, as workplace environment and safety are also critical concerns. Care should be based on the best evidence possible. Figure 3-1 presents this model, describing the interrelatedness of quality, evidence, and safety with the important guides such as standards, rules and regulations, policies and procedures, and others.

The standards provide significant background information to expand on and support the standards. Standards are "authoritative statements of the duties that all registered nurses, regardless of role, population, or specialty, are expected to perform competently" (ANA 2015c, 51). ANA has two types of standards that apply to all registered nurses (RNs). The first are called the Standards of Professional Nursing Practice. The Standards of Professional Nursing Practice focus on competent levels of nursing care applied in the nursing process, which emphasize critical thinking. It is also important to apply clinical reasoning and judgment along with critical

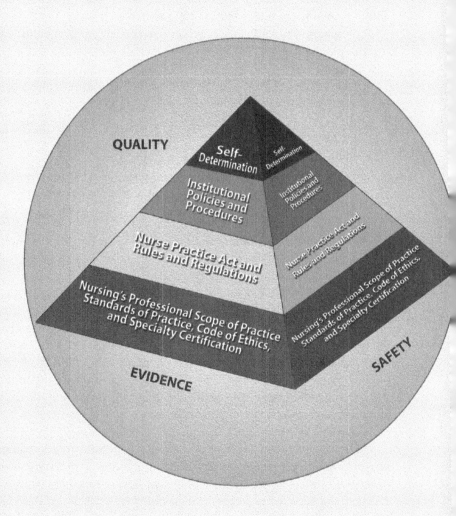

Model of Professional Nursing Practice Regulation

QUALITY

Self-Determination

Institutional Policies and Procedures

Nurse Practice Act and Rules and Regulations

Nursing's Professional Scope of Practice Standards of Practice, Code of Ethics, and Specialty Certification

EVIDENCE

SAFETY

Source note: This is a revision of a model published first in ANA, 2006, then revised in Styles, Schumann, Bickford, & White, 2008; ANA 2010a.

© 2015 American Nurses Association

FIGURE 3-1. **Model of Professional Nursing Practice Regulation**
   Source: American Nurses Association. 2015. *Nursing: Scope and Standards of Practice.* 3rd ed. Silver Spring, MD: Author.

Serif *text denotes the "what" of each tier.* Sans serif *text denotes the "who" of each tier.*

Peak: Self-Determination

This peak represents self-regulation and self-determination by each individual nurse in exercising judgments based upon the integration of content, decisions, and actions from the three lower tiers. The resultant demonstrated behaviors reflect responsible and accountable nursing practice decisions culminating in safe, quality, evidence-based practice. The peak culminates in a point directed upward synonymous to an illuminating path from Nightingale's lamp to emphasize continued potential toward a higher level of individual professional practice regulation.

Participants: Registered nurses, graduate-level prepared registered nurses, and advanced practice registered nurses*.

Institutional Policies and Procedures

Regulation at the institutional, organizational, or systems level occurs through the established policies, procedures, and governing statements that influence and direct nursing practice and its environment.

Participants: Institutions, organizations, entities, and systems where nurses are present, chief nursing officers and executives, healthcare administrators, nursing managers, nursing supervisors, registered nurses, graduate-level prepared registered nurses, advanced practice registered nurses*, third-party reimbursement entities, and academic institutions.

Nurse Practice Act and Rules and Regulations

Legislative and regulatory authorities govern through nurse practice acts, statute, code, and regulation administrated by state boards of nursing and exemplified by licensure status.

Participants: State or territorial boards of nursing, legislators, lobbyists, National Council of State Boards of Nursing, healthcare advocacy groups, healthcare consumers as voters, political action committees, registered nurses, graduate-leve prepared registered nurses, and advanced practice registered nurses.

Foundation: Nursing's Professional Scope of Practice, Standards of Practice, Code of Ethics, and Specialty Certification

ANA's *Nursing: Scope and Standards of Practice* and *Code of Ethics for Nurses with Interpretive Statements* are essential professional resources that collectively guide nursing practice in all roles and settings. Compliance with the *Code of Ethics for Nurses with Interpretive Statements* and identified standards of practice and accompanying competencies reflects the expected level of competence of all nurses. Specialty certification provides additional verification and validation of competence for a focused body of knowledge and associated skill sets of practice.

Participants: American Nurses Association, credentialing and educational organizations, professional nursing organizations, healthcare consumers as care partners, registered nurses, graduate-level prepared registered nurses, and advanced practice registered nurses*.

*(*The APRN direct care roles include certified registered nurse anesthetists, certified nurse midwives, clinical nurse specialists, and certified nurse practitioners.)*

thinking. These standards relate to the following aspects of practice and the nursing process (ANA 2015c, 53–66):

Standard 1. Assessment.

Standard 2. Diagnosis.

Standard 3. Outcomes Identification.

Standard 4. Planning.

Standard 5. Implementation.

5A. Coordination of Care.

5B. Health Teaching and Health Promotion.

Standard 6. Evaluation.

The second type of standards are the Standards of Professional Performance, which describe "a competent level of behavior in the professional role, including activities related to ethics, culturally congruent practice, communication, collaboration, leadership, education, evidence-based practice and research, quality of practice, professional practice evaluation, resource utilization, and environmental health" (ANA 2015c, 5). All of these issues are related to the *Quality Chasm* work on health care quality as described in chapter 1.

The Essential Guide to Nursing Practice: Applying ANA's Scope and Standards in Practice and Education provides additional examination of the application of the ANA's scope and standards of practice and education (White and O'Sullivan 2012). The ANA guide connects the social policy statement and regulation with the standards, providing examples and cases to illustrate application.

Code of Ethics for Nurses with Interpretive Statements (2015)

The *Code of Ethics for Nurses* (Fowler 2015a) is the third in the triad of critical ANA publications that forms a framework for the practice of nursing. The social policy statement and the standards require an ethical professional approach to health care. The *Code of Ethics for Nurses with Interpretive Statements* ("the Code") itself may be described as (1) a succinct statement of the ethical values, obligations, duties, and professional ideals of nurses individually and collectively; (2) the profession's nonnegotiable ethical standards; and (3) an expression of nursing's own understanding of its commitment to society (ANA 2015a, xiii). The Code, which applies to all nurses in the United States in all health care settings, includes nine provisions. Related core competencies are identified for each provision (ANA 2015a, v).

> "*Provision 1:* The nurse practices with compassion and respect for the inherent dignity, worth, and unique attributes of every person." Relates to the core competency of patient-centered care, which includes diversity concerns.

> "*Provision 2:* The nurse's primary commitment is to the patient, whether an individual, family, group, community, or population." Relates to the core competency of patient-centered care.

> "*Provision 3:* The nurse promotes, advocates for, and protects the rights, health, and safety of the patient." Relates to the core competencies of patient-centered care and quality improvement.

> "*Provision 4:* The nurse has authority, accountability, and responsibility for nursing practice; makes decisions; and takes action consistent with the obligation to promote health and to provide optimal care." Relates to the core competencies of patient-centered care and interprofessional teamwork.

> "*Provision 5:* The nurse owes the same duties to self as to others, including the responsibility to preserve integrity and safety, to maintain competence, and to continue personal and professional growth." Relates to the core competency of quality improvement.

> "*Provision 6:* The nurse, through individual and collective effort, establishes, maintains, and improves the ethical environment of the work setting and conditions of employment that are conducive to safe, quality health care." Relates to the core competencies of quality improvement, interprofessional teamwork, evidence-based practice, and informatics.

> "*Provision 7:* The nurse, in all roles and settings, advances the profession through research and scholarly inquiry, professional standards development, and the generation of both nursing and health policy." Relates to the core competencies of quality improvement and evidence-based practice or management.

> "*Provision 8:* The nurse collaborates with other health professionals and the public to protect human rights, promote health diplomacy, and reduce health disparities." Relates to the core competencies of patient-centered care and interprofessional teamwork.

> "*Provision 9:* The profession of nursing, collectively through its professional organizations, must articulate nursing values, maintain the integrity of the profession, and integrate principles of social justice into nursing and health policy." Relates to the core competency of quality improvement.

Trossman (2011) discusses the role of the nurse-ethicist, describing it as a nurse who teaches about ethics, provides formal ethics consults, and discusses ethical concerns with nurses informally. Every nurse makes ethical decisions every day, even if it is just to decide who gets care first. This does not mean that there is always an ethical conflict in these decisions. How should you integrate the Code into your daily practice? Another ANA publication, *Guide to the Code of Ethics for Nurses with Interpretive Statements* (Fowler 2015a), expands on the Code, providing additional resources and examples.

Nursing Administration: Scope and Standards of Practice (2016)

Nursing Administration: Scope and Standards of Practice, 2nd edition, contains important standards that focus on the intersection of administration and nursing in all settings. Since we are in a period of greater emphasis on leadership as commented on in *The Future of Nursing* (IOM 2011a) report, there is more concern about the quality of care, which requires administration and staff working to resolve quality problems and improve care and services. Major changes in reimbursement and other health care delivery changes due to the passage of the Affordable Care Act (ACA) of 2010 was also increasing the need for nursing administration standards. The standards of practice for nursing administration are (ANA 2016e, 35–43):

Standard 1. Assessment. The nurse-administrator collects pertinent data and information relative to the situation, issue, problem, or trend.

Standard 2. Identification of Problems, Issues, and Trends. The nurse-administrator analyzes the assessment data to identify problems, issues, and trends.

Standard 3. Outcomes Identification. The nurse-administrator identifies expected outcomes for a plan tailored to the system, organization, or population problem, issue, or trend.

Standard 4. Planning. The nurse-administrator develops a plan that defines, articulates, and establishes strategies and alternatives to attain expected, measurable outcomes.

Standard 5. Implementation. The nurse-administrator implements the identified plan.

Standard 5A. Coordination. The nurse-administrator coordinates implementation of the plan and associated processes.

Standard 5B. Promotion of Health, Education, and a Safe Environment. The nurse-administrator establishes strategies to promote health, education, and a safe environment.

Standard 6. Evaluation. The nurse-administrator evaluates progress toward the attainment of goals and outcomes.

In addition to the standards for nursing administration practice are the standards for the professional performance of nurses in this field. They are (ANA 2016e, 45–59):

Standard 7. Ethics. The nurse administrator practices ethically.

Standard 8. Culturally Congruent Practice. The nurse administrator practices in a safe manner that is congruent with cultural diversity and inclusion principles.

Standard 9. Communication. The nurse administrator communicates effectively in all areas of practice.

Standard 10. Collaboration. The nurse administrator collaborates with the health care consumer and other key stakeholders in the conduct of nursing practice.

Standard 11. Leadership. The nurse administrator leads within the professional practice setting, profession, health care industry, and society.

Standard 12. Education. The nurse administrator seeks knowledge and competence that reflect current nursing practice and promotes futuristic thinking.

Standard 13. Evidence-based Practice and Research. The nurse administrator integrates evidence and research findings into practice.

Standard 14. Quality of Practice. The nurse administrator contributes to quality nursing practice.

Standard 15. Professional Practice Evaluation. The nurse administrator evaluates one's own and others' nursing practice.

Standard 16. Resource Utilization. The nurse administrator utilizes appropriate resources to plan, provide, and sustain high quality nursing services that are person-, population-, or community-centered, culturally appropriate, safe, effective, and fiscally responsible.

Standard 17. Environmental Health. The nurse administrator practices in an environmentally safe and healthy manner.

These published standards provide supporting information about nursing administration and need for standards in this specialty area. Nursing administration is the "specialty practice devoted to the design, facilitation, supervision, and evaluation of systems that educate and/or employ nurses" (ANA 2016e, 2). Nurse-administrators work in a variety of setting and roles in practice and in education.

Nursing Informatics: Scope and Standards of Practice (2015)

Nursing Informatics: Scope and Standards of Practice, 2nd edition, provides important practice and professional performance standards at a time when we are expanding health informatics technology (HIT). This area is also one of the five core health care profession competencies—utilize informatics. Beyond the more general need for all nurses to have an understanding of HIT and participate in its use, nursing informatics is a specialty that "integrates nursing science with multiple information and analytical sciences to identify, define, manage, and communicate data, information, knowledge, and wisdom in nursing practice" (ANA 2015b, 1-2). In this specialty nurses hold a variety of positions in many different health care settings. The published standards provide extensive background information about informatics and also technology in health care and related issues such as regulation. The standards of nursing informatics practice include the following (ANA 2015b, 68-78):

> **Standard 1. Assessment.** The informatics nurse collects comprehensive data, information, and emerging evidence pertinent to the situation.
>
> **Standard 2. Diagnosis, Problems, Issues Identification.** The informatics nurse analyzes assessment data to identify diagnoses, problems, issues, and opportunities for improvement.
>
> **Standard 3. Outcomes Identification.** The informatics nurse identifies expected outcomes for a plan individualized to the health care consumer or the situation.
>
> **Standard 4. Planning.** The informatics nurse develops a plan that prescribes strategies, alternatives, and recommendations to attain expected outcomes.
>
> **Standard 5. Implementation.** The informatics nurse implements the identified plan.
>
>> *Standard 5a. Coordination of Activities.* The informatics nurse coordinates planned activities.
>>
>> *Standard 5b. Health Teaching and Health Promotion.* The informatics nurse employs informatics solutions and strategies for education and teaching to promote health and a safe environment.

Standard 5c. Consultation. The informatics nurse provides consultation to influence the identified plan, enhance the abilities of others, and effect change.

Standard 6. Evaluation. The informatics nurse evaluates progress toward attainment of outcomes.

In addition to the standards for nursing informatics practice are the standards for the professional performance of nurses in this field (ANA 2015b, 70–94):

Standard 7. Ethics. The informatics nurse practices ethically.

Standard 8. Education. The informatics nurse attains knowledge and competence that reflect current nursing and informatics practices.

Standard 9. Evidence-Based Practice and Research. The informatics nurse integrates evidence and research findings into practice.

Standard 10. Quality of Practice. The informatics nurse contributes to the quality and effectiveness of nursing and informatics practice.

Standard 11. Communication. The informatics nurse communicates effectively in a variety of formats in all areas of practice.

Standard 12. Leadership. The informatics nurse demonstrates leadership in the professional practice setting and the profession.

Standard 13. Collaboration. The informatics nurse collaborates with the health care consumer, family, and others in the conduct of nursing and informatics practice.

Standard 14. Professional Practice Evaluation. The informatics nurse evaluates his or her own nursing practice in relation to professional practice standards and guidelines, relevant statutes, rules, and regulations.

Standard 15. Resource Utilization. The informatics nurse employs appropriate resources to plan and implement informatics and associated services that are safe, effective, and fiscally responsible.

Standard 16. Environmental Health. The informatics nurse supports practice in a safe and healthy environment.

Nursing Professional Development: Scope and Standards of Practice (2016)

The standards that focus on staff development and other areas of nursing professional development are included in *Nursing Professional Development: Scope and Standards of Practice* 3rd Edition (ANPD 2016). Published by the Association for Nursing Professional Development, a leading professional organization in this specialty, it was developed with and approved by ANA. These standards are grounded in the same criteria and core documents as the current editions of *Nursing: Scope and Standards of Practice* and *Nursing Informatics: Scope and Standards of Practice.*

In addition, these standards and current nursing professional development (NPD) practice clearly reflects several of the IOM interprofessional competencies as well as aspects and concerns of the *Quality Chasm* and other reports. This is evident in the NPD Specialist Practice Model (ANPD 2016, 10), shown in figure 3-2, which illustrates the essentials of NPD practice and features such core responsibilities as evidence-based practice, quality improvement, and interprofessional collaboration.

The NPD-specific perspective on interprofessional practice in this model (ANPD 2016, 9) expands on this element:

> *All NPD activities occur in the context of interprofessional practice and learning environments. The NPD practitioner and learner operate in these two environments that have fluid and evolving boundaries. The NPD practice environment may overlap with the learner's environment.*

This viewpoint exemplifies the practice–education balance that is needed throughout nursing. This imperative threads through the IOM/HMD reports that are summarized in this book, and each edition of this book. More dialogue, more collaboration, more partnering among nurses, particularly nurses in education and nurses in practice.

Other critical elements of the model's process are staff education, role development, and competency management. In the NPD model, learning includes both continuing education for nurses and interprofessional education (ANPD 2016, 18) along with professional role competence and growth—is directly linked to optimal care and health outcomes. As is true for all of the nursing standards developed by and with ANA, this reflects ANA's view on nursing's essential social concerns and social contract to provide quality care and protect the public.

Summing Up: Key Nursing Documents and the IOM/HMD Reports

Combining these policy and practice documents—nursing's social policy statement, some of its key standards, and its code of ethics—with the IOM/HMD in-depth examinations and published reports on the health care

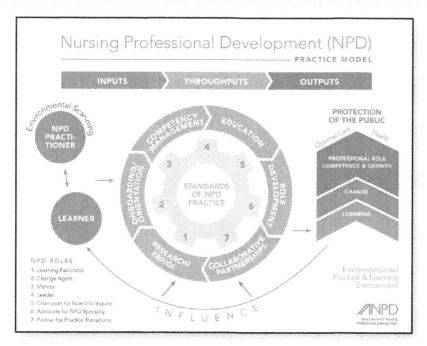

FIGURE 3-2. **Nursing Professional Development Practice Model**
Source: Harper, M. G., and P. Maloney, eds. 2016. *Nursing Professional Development: Scope and Standards of Practice*. 3rd ed. Chicago, IL: Association for Nursing Professional Development. Reprinted with permission from the Association for Nursing Professional Development.

system, quality improvement, and the core competencies required for improvement provides students and nurses with a strong framework within which to develop as a professional. As noted in *The Future of Nursing*, the large number of nurses is a strength of the profession that can help increase nursing's ability to participate and even to lead in health care change. With the profession's knowledge of and experience with care across the continuum and working with teams and other health care professionals in all types of settings, nurses can make a difference now and as the delivery system changes and improves (IOM 2011a). This effort requires nursing competence, leadership, and engagement in quality improvement.

Part II

Incorporating the Core Competencies into Nursing Education

The strategies for integrating quality care content and experiences in nursing education are based on the five core competencies found in *Health Professions Education* (Greiner and Knebel 2003):

- Provide patient-centered care
- Work in interprofessional teams
- Employ evidence-based practice
- Apply quality improvement
- Utilize informatics

The *Quality Chasm* reports include significant reforms. There has been a shift to a competency-based approach to education for all health care professions. The core competencies identified are essential for health care professionals to respond effectively to patients' care needs. "It is tempting to say we already do these things (five core competencies). Surely we have been talking about informatics competencies for a long time, and we expect our graduates to be leaders and to work in interdisciplinary [inter-professional] teams....It is now time to work toward building one bridge over the quality chasm" (Tanner 2003, 432).

Figure 4-1 describes the connection between the initial reports in the *Quality Chasm* series and the health care professions core competencies. This part of the book discusses content and strategies for each of the core competencies.

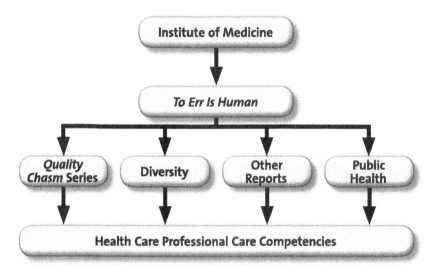

FIGURE 4-1. **Development of the IOM health care core competencies**
Source: National Council of State Boards of Nursing. 2013. "Meeting the Ongoing Challenge of Continued Competence." https://www.ncsbn.org/Continued_Comp_Paper_TestingServices.pdf. Reproduced with permission of NCSBN.

4

Core Competency: Provide Patient-Centered Care

*Identify, respect, and care about patients' differ-
ences, values, preferences, and expressed needs;
relieve pain and suffering; coordinate continuous
care; listen to, clearly inform, communicate with,
and educate patients; share decision-making
and management; and continuously advocate
disease prevention, wellness, and promotion of
healthy lifestyles, including a focus on population health.* (Greiner and Knebel 2003, 4)

Patient-centered care (PCC) puts the focus on the patient and family
instead of on health care professionals; for example, one approach to
emphasizing PCC in practice might be to have the health care professionals
come to the patient instead of moving the patient from room to room to
see different specialists. All health care professionals should be educated
to deliver PCC as members of an interprofessional team, emphasizing
evidence-based practice (EBP), quality improvement (QI) approaches, and
health informatics technology (HIT) (Greiner and Knebel 2003). Nursing
education must adapt to the changing demographics of the patient population, integrate new technologies, and meet critical competencies. The
following content describes some of the issues related to PCC that should
be considered in nursing and staff education.

Decentralized and Fragmented Care

You may have experienced fragmented care with your patients but may not have recognized it. If you do not recognize it, you may often be frustrated by it. How did it feel when you first entered the health care setting as a student? Some common reactions are confusion, inability to understand what is going on, uncertainty as to who staff are and what the expectations are, unclear communication, and so on. Considering this experience can help you better appreciate what patients may be feeling. When a test is delayed or postponed because someone did not order it, how does the patient feel and react, and what impact does this have on patient care when the you well-planned schedule for care is no longer well planned? The goal is for you to better appreciate the trajectory or course of illness and the continuum of care.

Fragmented care exists throughout the health care system. Can you think of examples of fragmented care and their practical solutions? Iatrogenic injury can be related to fragmented care. How might this occur in different health care settings, such as acute care, emergency department (ED), ambulatory care, and home care?

What are the implications of decentralization and fragmentation on the nursing process? This discussion has two sides. Decentralization allows decision-making to be made closer to the patient and reinforces more autonomy at lower levels of an organization, but it can lead to variations in care from unit to unit and fragmentation of services. Consider how plans of care might ensure more decentralization and less fragmentation to improve safety. What might be the role of the nurse in that effort?

Self-Management Support

Self-management support is "the systematic provision of education and supportive interventions to increase patients' skills and confidence in managing their health problems, including regular assessment of progress and problems, goal setting, and problem-solving support" (Adams and Corrigan 2003, 52). Another term for self-management is *self-care*. Self-management is particularly important in chronic illnesses, such as diabetes and asthma, and becomes even more complex when patients have multiple problems. Self-management is an appropriate means to assist patients who have acute care problems with returning to their usual daily functioning as soon as possible; it is also a critical component of care for patients with chronic illnesses, as is care coordination. Self-management support and care coordination should be integral parts of nursing care, and with the added emphasis on them, nurses should be taking a greater lead in research about self-management and developing effective interventions for patients and families or significant others. You should consider self-management for every patient you care for and include the patient and the patient's family in the process. It is important to note you must follow the patient's view on informing his or her family, what can be shared, and how family should participate.

Effective self-management support requires collaboration between the patient and all providers involved in the care. This support requires services such as improving and supporting patient and family confidence in their role and in the care process; providing effective patient and family education about health and care; recognizing and accepting patient preferences; and meeting psychosocial and medical needs (Institute for Health Improvement 2008a). Even patients with acute illnesses can benefit from more effective self-management.

Patient Errors in Self-Management

Although self-management allows patients to be more independent, it can also lead to errors. How can we help patients avoid errors during self-management? Patients at risk for self-management errors include those with multiple chronic problems using multiple medications and elderly patients trying to practice self-management in their homes. You can help patients with self-management by knowing how to assist them in using Medisets to administer their medication; how to monitor medication use by patients and caregivers; and how to teach patients and caregivers what to review when they receive or give medications, such as drug name and dose. Consider how confusing multiple oral medications with complex administration schedules might be for patients, and if patients can open childproof lids and read small-print labels (e.g., in cases of arthritis, poor eyesight, etc.). How easy is it for a patient to make an error? What methods can you use to educate patients and their families, prevent errors, and help them improve their self-management? Medication reconciliation, which is discussed later, is also highly relevant to self-management.

Disease Management and Patient-Centered Care

Disease management, which involves self-management, can help decrease complications, length of stay, and costs. Effective disease management involves care coordination, interprofessional teamwork, and patient-centered care. Patients who can particularly benefit include those who are chronically or critically ill. Nurse or patient navigation is used in some clinical settings to assist patients through their treatment trajectory to meet their health needs. The nurse navigator works with the patient and family to guide them through the complex health care system to ensure better outcomes. Advanced practice registered nurses (APRNs) and clinical nurse leaders (CNLs) often serve in this role.

The goals of disease management are to improve quality of life, decrease disease progression, and reduce hospitalizations and rehospitalizations. A nurse call center typically provides services such as monitoring health status, providing patient education and advice, and sharing information from physicians, medical labs, and pharmacies. Chronic illnesses that are typically monitored include diabetes, heart disease and hypertension, asthma, cancer, depression, renal disease, low back pain, and obesity. Insurers typically develop disease management programs and use case management to control costs (Finkelman 2011). Content on disease management and also case management can be included in public and community health content and experiences. Planning care for these patients requires incorporation of the following patient needs:

- Understand basic information about their disease. (Even if the patient already has this information, you should confirm patient retention and understanding and be prepared to share or review this information as needed or requested.)
- Understand the importance of self-management and development of skills required to effectively self-manage care.
- Recognize the need for ongoing support from members of the practice team, family, friends, and community.

The Institute for Healthcare Improvement (IHI) offers tools to support self-management on its website (http://www.ihi.org/resources/Pages/Changes/SelfManagement.aspx). Examples of the tools are: Quality Compass Benchmarks, Blood Pressure Visual Aid for Patients, Self-Management Support: Patient Planning Worksheet, My Shared Plan, and Group Visit Starter Kit.

Chronic Disease and Self-Management

The number of persons with chronic diseases has increased, as has the number of people with more than one chronic disease. Some data on chronic disease include (CDC 2016b):

- As of 2012, about half of all adults had one or more chronic health conditions.

- In 2010, seven of the ten leading causes of death were chronic diseases.
- Obesity has become a major health concern for children and adults.
- High-risk behaviors that cause chronic diseases continue, such as drinking too much alcohol, smoking, and insufficient exercise.
- In 2010, 86 percent of all health care spending was for care of people with one or more chronic disease(s).

Why does the United States have these problems with chronic disease? One reason is that with the better treatment available today people with chronic diseases live longer; consequently, there are more of them. The United States must improve care provided for those with chronic diseases (https://www.cdc.gov/chronicdisease/index.htm). Many of the priority areas of care, monitored annually in the National Healthcare Quality and Disparities Report (QDR), are chronic diseases.

Effective management of a chronic illness requires daily management of the illness but also should include activities to improve health in general. To accomplish this, the person with chronic illness needs to have an understanding of the illness and the interventions in order to achieve self-management, focusing on care of the body and management of the condition, adapting everyday activities and roles to the condition, and dealing with emotions arising from having the condition.

The Chronic Care Model is a patient-centered approach applied in some clinical settings. It can also be used to guide you in understanding chronic illness (http://www.improvingchroniccare.org/; Wagner 1998; Improving Chronic Illness Care 2003). The model emphasizes two principles:

1. The *community* should have resources and health policies that support care for chronic illnesses.
2. The *health system* should include health care organizations (HCOs) that support self-management, recognizing that the patient is the source of control (patient-centered); a delivery system design that identifies clear roles for staff in relationship to chronic illness care; decision support with evidence-based guidelines integrated into daily practice; and clinical information systems to ensure rapid exchange of information and reminder and feedback systems.

This model can be found at the Improving Chronic Illness Care website (http://www.improvingchroniccare.org; IHI 2016c). This site offers graphics and information about this topic, including links to content, links to content, application of the model to care issues, and audiovisual presentations.

Self-Management and Diversity

How do cultural issues affect self-management? How is the community involved? When providing care for chronic illness, the community is important as this is where most of the prevention of chronic illness and care for chronic illness occurs. Patients from different ethnic groups may respond to chronic illness and to self-management differently. Language affects patients' abilities to understand directions, which is critical to effective self-management. Family roles vary in different cultures, which can influence how families respond and the roles they may or may not assume. Healthy literacy (discussed later) is a critical factor in ensuring quality care in any diversity situation.

Diversity and Disparities in Health Care

Diversity and disparities in health care are critical components of PCC—affecting patient needs and responses, communication, quality, and outcomes throughout the continuum of care. Disparities can be a difficult topic for faculty and students. Health care providers view themselves as caring, open people. You need opportunities to discuss cultural issues in a safe environment—one in which opinions will not be negatively criticized, but rather will be used to develop professional attitudes and behaviors. For example, you need to understand that patients may mistrust the health care system because they have experienced bias from health care providers in the past. Communication is a critical element, and health literacy also plays a major role in disparities. Cultural competence is also highly personal. Take some time to consider your own cultural background and how this influences you personally and might influence your practice. Several topics in this chapter provide information about this issue in health care and also relate back to reports summarized in part 1.

Reacting to the Shifting Demographics of the Patient Population

Americans are older than ever, living longer with multiple comorbidities and chronic health needs. The other end of the life span is also at increasing risk, with a population of children who before the age of ten experiencing comorbidities such as hypertension, diabetes, and obesity; furthermore, many women are delaying childbearing into their forties, which may lead to complications during pregnancy and for the newborn.

These demographics indicate that long-term health care requires a delivery system capable of handling this growing complexity. Because these are dramatic shifts away from the patient pool of the past, health care professionals need education that prepares them to intervene in complex health problems in a more efficient, safe way to reach quality outcomes that are also cost-effective. The goal is for practicing nurses to recognize the relevance of and integrate cultural factors and needs in care planning and delivery.

At the same time, the population is becoming more diverse. Understanding cultural beliefs and values and their relationship to each other are part of developing cultural competence. Understanding the demographics and cultural backgrounds of your patients and addressing them in patient care plans is an important part of providing care to diverse populations.

Emergency Care and Diversity and Disparities

Emergency care is a critical concern in the United States, as noted in the *Quality Chasm reports on emergency medical services discussed in* chapter 1. A common assumption is that we have this problem because so many uninsured persons use the ED when they do not need emergency care. Actually, this is not correct. After the Affordable Care Act (ACA) was implemented, an update of the data on use of emergency services indicated there was little change from 2013 to 2014 (Gindi, Black, and Cohen 2016): In 2014, 18 percent of adults visited the ED one or more times. For 77 percent of adults aged 18–64, the seriousness of the medical problem was the reason for the most recent ED visit; 12 percent went because their doctor's office was not open; and 7 percent went because of a lack of access to other providers (4 percent did not select any reason). Percentages were similar in 2013.

Controlling for other variables, adults with Medicaid coverage were most likely to report that seriousness of the medical problem was the reason for the most recent ED visit. Adults with private coverage were most likely to have used the ED because the doctor's office was not open. Uninsured adults were more likely than adults with private coverage to have visited the ED because they lacked access to other providers. Differences in reasons for use between demographic groups were also identified. The Centers for Disease Control and Prevention (CDC) website (https://www.cdc.gov/) provides current data on the use of all types of health care services, such as emergency services.

Diversity issues are prevalent in emergency care, and the need for quick, effective communication with patients and families is critical. Accessibility of interpreters is often a barrier in the emergency care delivery system.

Emergency departments have the only legal mandate in the US health care system to provide health care, according to the Emergency Medical Treatment and Labor Act (EMTALA). This law ensures that anyone who comes to an ED, regardless of their insurance status or ability to pay, must receive a medical screening exam and be stabilized.

Patients with nonurgent medical conditions may wait longer to be seen, but once seen, they should be treated quickly and released. Many EDs experience routine or occasional patient overflow problems, which may be due to lack of hospital resources such as staff, ED space, and limited access to inpatient beds (American College of Emergency Physicians [ACEP] 2011). Several of the Health and Medicine Division (HMD) reports on emergency care comment on this problem, as described in chapter 1.

Clinical Trials and Disparities

The current design and administration of clinical trials in the United States underrepresents certain populations such as African Americans, Hispanic Americans, women, and older Americans (Mozes 2008). Mozes's study indicates that the disparities are largely due to reliance on strict sample inclusion or exclusion criteria, the use of lengthy and complicated consent forms available only in English, and a lack of specific information on cost reimbursement for participants. These disparities can skew treatment recommendations that are based on studies with inequitable representation in their samples. We need to expand clinical trial participation so research results can better reflect all populations. *Sharing Clinical Trial Data: Maximizing Benefits, Minimizing Risk* (HMD 2015b) provides some current perspectives on clinical trials.

Evidence-based practice (EBP) should also consider diversity as an important factor in determining best evidence (Minority Nurse Staff 2008). Because many studies do not include racially diverse participants, it is critical to determine similarities or differences in populations when reviewing evidence to better ensure effective EBP. This content is relevant to nursing research courses and all courses that integrate EBP.

Disparities in Rural Areas

Typically, care for people who live in rural areas is covered in public and community health content. The rural population often includes multiple ethnic groups, but the rural population as a whole also experiences disparities in health care due to risk factors such as higher incidence of disease and disability, increased mortality rates, lower life expectancies, and higher rates for pain and suffering (Rural Health Information Hub [RHIHub] 2016). Examples of differences in health problems from urban areas are higher rates of ischemic heart disease, unintentional injury, suicide, teen births, preventable hospital admissions, diabetes, activity limitation due to chronic disease, and others. Rural areas have problems attracting and retaining health care professionals and may struggle with keeping hospitals financially viable. Transportation to health services is also a problem along with economic issues that may lead to unemployment and an increased number of uninsured.

Much more must be done to improve care in rural areas. The National Rural Health Association (NRHA) website provides important current information on this topic (https://www.ruralhealthweb.org/).

Diversity and The Joint Commission

The Joint Commission offers a practical guide that HCOs can use to develop and improve programs and services to accommodate the needs of diverse populations. It recommends that HCO leadership instill concern for diverse patients, which should be demonstrated through policies and procedures; participation in ongoing data collection about patient culture and language needs; provision of care that meets diverse needs and related patient education; and collaboration with the local community in developing plans to meet cultural needs (Wilson-Stronks et al. 2008). A report titled *Advancing Effective Communication, Cultural Competence, and Patient- and Family-Centered Care: A Roadmap for Hospitals* is available online, along with other Joint Commission resources on diverse patient populations (Wilson-Stronks et al. 2010).

The National Healthcare Quality and Disparities Report

As mentioned in chapter 1, there is a pressing need to monitor health care disparities (Swift 2002). The annual QDR is available at the Agency Healthcare Research and Quality (AHRQ) website. The current report focuses on three questions (AHRQ 2015):

1. What is the status of health care quality and disparities in the United States?
2. How have health care quality and disparities changed over time?
3. Where is the need to improve health care quality and reduce disparities greatest?

Now the National Healthcare Quality and Disparities reports are combined into one report, the QDR. The annual report provides an excellent tool for students to understand current health care issues by reviewing the report's data.

The QDR is connected to the report *Healthy People in Healthy Communities* (Guidry et al. 2010), and to the Healthy People initiative—figure 4-2 describes the *Healthy People 2020* framework. This content relates to public and community health.

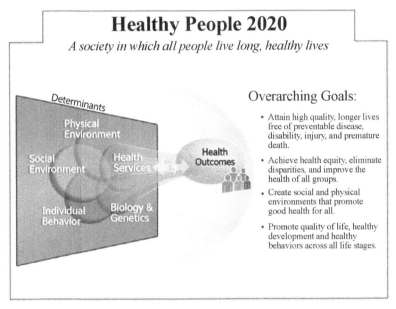

FIGURE 4-2. *Healthy People 2020 framework*
Source: Office of Disease Prevention and Health Promotion. N.d. "*Healthy People 2020* Framework." https://www.healthypeople.gov/sites/default/files/HP2020Framework.pdf

Cultural Competence

A paper from American Association of Colleges of Nursing (AACN) describes background and content that should be considered in baccalaureate programs to facilitate cultural competence (AACN 2008a). This document complements *The Essentials of Baccalaureate Education for Professional Nursing Practice*. The AACN cultural competence toolkit identifies five competencies for culturally competent care and content recommendations. The competencies focus on knowledge of social and cultural factors, importance of data and evidence, safe and quality outcomes, advocacy of social justice, and participation in development of cultural competence (AACN 2008a, 2008c).

In 2011, the AACN published *Tool Kit for Cultural Competence in Master's and Doctoral Nursing Education*, available on its website (AACN 2011b) and a number of other resources for various nursing programs.

Another definition of *cultural competence* is the "attitudes, knowledge, and skills necessary for providing quality care to diverse populations" (California Endowment 2003, as cited in AACN 2008b, 1). Cultural competence is not just relevant to prelicensure nursing programs but also to graduate programs, for example *The Essentials of Master's Education* also emphasizes the need for cultural competence in Essential VIII, which notes that the master's-prepared nurse "applies and integrates broad, organizational, client-centered, and *culturally appropriate* concepts in the planning, delivery, management, and evaluation of evidence-based clinical prevention and population care and services to individuals, families, and aggregates/identified populations" (AACN 2011a, 5).

Health Literacy

Health literacy is "the ability to read, understand, and act on health care information" (Nielsen-Bohlman, Panzer, and Kindig 2004, 52). You need to learn how to assess patient understanding and to make changes in care as required. There are many examples of medical forms and brochures that are supposed to provide patients with information, but the information is not always easy to understand, even for people whose first language is English. The Joint Commission's accreditation standards emphasize the importance of health literacy in HCOs and provide methods to integrate health literacy to better ensure that cultural needs are met (The Joint Commission 2007).

An investigation of the relationship between health literacy and adherence to clinical outcomes reviewed 44 studies (DeWalt et al. 2004). This review notes that people with lower health literacy tended to have more adverse outcomes. The review also notes that there is a greater chance of Medicare enrollees with lower literacy never receiving prevention screening (e.g., a Pap smear, a mammogram, etc.) or influenza and pneumococcal immunizations, and having an increased risk for hospitalization as compared to enrollees with greater health literacy.

Health illiteracy is more common in vulnerable populations such as low-income or racial and ethnic minorities (Ferguson 2008). Women influence the health of children because women are usually the caregivers. If a woman's health literacy is low, this puts her children at risk. Pregnant women who do not understand health information can affect the fetus and the infant's health and development after birth (Puchner 1995; Ferguson 2008). The major barriers to quality health care associated with health literacy are inability to access care (e.g., insurance, availability of health care providers, appointments, etc.), manage illness (e.g., complicated problems and treatment, multiple health care providers who may not always agree, patient-provider communication), and process information (e.g., informed consent, privacy and confidentiality, access to care information, confusion about health care bills) (DeWalt and Pignone 2008).

Patient advocacy can make a major difference in helping patients and families who are experiencing health literacy problems (http://www.ahrq.gov/patients-consumers/index.html). One of the goals of *Healthy People 2020* is to improve consumer health literacy. The Food and Drug Administration (FDA) has also made changes to regulate drug information and improve health literacy. A good source illustrating the importance of labeling and health literacy is the American College of Physicians Foundation's (2007) white paper on drug container labeling. Limited health literacy leads to higher outpatient medication errors, possible adverse events and complications, increased costs, and an inability to reach positive outcomes.

Health Literacy and Self-Management

Self-management will not be effective if the patient has a low level of health literacy. Why is this the case? What skills do patients need to manage their diabetes or arthritis? Consider how health literacy problems might relate to adult health, pediatrics, mental health, obstetrics, and public and community health. Nurses need to understand that health literacy issues can arise in all health care situations and have an impact on care and outcomes.

What does health literacy mean to you? How does your view of health literacy compare to the definition of health literacy? Try to imagine the stigma that health-illiterate patients may feel.

Using Interpreters

Have you ever worked with an interpreter to facilitate communication with a patient? It can be a frustrating experience trying to communicate through a third party. Make sure you speak directly to the patient, even though the natural tendency is to speak to the interpreter. What might be the advantages and disadvantages of depending on family members as interpreters? What might be the impact on a female patient of a culture in which the husband makes decisions? Would the wife feel comfortable expressing herself, and would the husband try to soften difficult messages and then make decisions for the wife, the patient? Would it be better to use a native speaker or a language expert to interpret? There are options if no interpreter is available, such as finding a health care provider who speaks the language, working with community groups to help interpret, preparing visual materials that might aid communication, and so on.

Health Literacy and the Health Care Delivery System

What is done in a specific HCO to address health literacy? How do health agencies used for clinical experiences respond to health literacy in their patient information and education programs? You can gather information by observation, interviewing staff, and reviewing written materials and other types of educational materials (such as videos that might be shown to patients). Are interpreters available and are they used? Is hearing-impaired equipment accessible and is it used? Look at signs and their effectiveness; for example, the use of colors to direct patients. What could be improved and how could the environment be changed so that all patients can be understood and better understand health care providers?

Health Literacy, Nursing Assessment, and Interventions

You can assess health literacy levels within a population group in your community or an agency and its patients, identify problems and interventions that were used and their outcomes; then consider other types of interventions that might improve health literacy. Health literacy should be part of individual patient assessments. Is health literacy included in your patient assessments? If not, how could it be included? How should this assessment be done? Is it part of an HCO's standard assessment forms? Compare assessment forms from different HCOs or different services within an HCO.

The AHRQ website offers information about health literacy measurement tools to assist care providers in assessing and providing the best solutions to improve health literacy (AHRQ 2016). Tools are provided in several languages. You can examine these tools and consider how you might use them with patients.

Pain Management

Pain is a major health care problem, with 116 million adults in the United States experiencing common chronic pain conditions, at a conservatively estimated annual cost of $560–$635 billion (IOM 2011c). This cost has undoubtedly risen since this report commented on the cost of pain management. In addition, *Healthy People 2020* recognizes the problem and includes an objective related to pain: increase the safe and effective treatment of pain. Health literacy is related to pain management. Many preventable adverse events are due to problems with understanding medication directions. There are also disparities in who receives effective treatment for pain, as discussed in the report on pain management (see Part I). Patient education is a critical intervention, and one that directly involves nurses, who have an important role in providing care for patients with pain; pain management is an essential responsibility of nurses. Nurses may also be involved in research to improve care for pain, particularly interprofessional research.

With the growing US opioid epidemic, the issue of pain management has become even more important. In 2016, the HHS increased funding for grants to address this critical problem. There is greater support now to use medications to treat opioid addiction and reduce overdose deaths (NIH 2014). The Obama administration identified key steps to be taken, such as preventing overdose, increasing parity in Medicaid for treatment of mental and substance use disorders, expanding partnerships to improve responses to use of heroin, addressing the problem actively in rural areas, creating a syringe use services program, and other responses (White House 2016). Nurses need more information and a better understanding of this problem, and they need to be involved in improving care to respond to it.

Pain management has long been a part of nursing curricula, though all nursing programs should review their content and placement of content to ensure that it is as up-to-date as possible. Pain management is a critical part of PCC. This pain management report is an excellent resource for students, providing background information on pain as well as viewing pain as a public health challenge and describing the picture of pain, identifying the many different types of people with pain (Figure 1-1, IOM 2011c, 27).

End-of-Life and Palliative Care

End-of-life and palliative care are two topics that are finding their way into more nursing curricula. *Quality Chasm* reports include these topics in the description of PCC and in a published a report called *Improving Palliative Care for Cancer: Summary and Recommendations* (Foley and Gelband 2001). This report is a good resource for students. According to this report, the health care system continues to underrecognize, underdiagnose, and undertreat patients who experience significant suffering from their illness. Palliative care is needed to focus on management of pain and other symptoms including psychological, social, and spiritual. To accomplish this, health care providers need to use effective communication and decision-making.

You need to understand these important aspects of care, the barriers to providing effective care, and interventions that can assist patients and families. You need to have an open dialogue about provider aspects of responses to patients who require this care as provider attitudes do make a difference in effective palliative care (Foley and Gelband 2001).

Patient Advocacy

Today, the patient is recognized as having a major role in efforts to reach positive health care outcomes and influence change in the health care delivery system (IOM 2007a, 25). It is difficult to discuss PCC without considering patient advocacy. A patient advocate or the patient navigator guides the patient in making informed decisions about health to reach best outcomes (Earp, French, and Gilkey 2008). Nurses describe themselves as patient advocates, but in the Earp, French, and Gilkey publication on patient advocacy there were no nurse authors or editors, and nursing is mentioned only in the beginning of the book. The book's content is based on content from a large conference on patient advocacy that was held in 2003 and 2005; it is notable that nursing did not have a leadership role. Today, more is being done to offer effective patient advocacy as part of PCC with more active nursing leadership—though much more is needed.

You need to understand patient advocacy, your own role, and strategies to improve advocacy. Patients can help teach you by explaining their illness and care experiences, helping create more effective patient teaching materials, and participating on health boards, advisory committees, and other types of health organizations, providing valuable input. You may have had patient experiences, either your own or a family member's. Consider these experiences when you examine patient advocacy.

Privacy, Confidentiality, and HIPAA

The topics of privacy, confidentiality, and the Health Insurance and Accountability Act (HIPAA) relate to PCC and should be introduced early in the curriculum when PCC is introduced. The critical issue is that *the patient makes decisions about his or her health care.* Health care providers share their expertise and recommendations, but do not make the decisions. A patient may decide to defer to the health care professional, but it should never be assumed that the patient will do so. You also need to clearly understand all aspects of patient information use and sharing. For example, consider the ramifications of electronic communication for patient privacy, such as the issue of taking photos with cell phones while in clinical areas and then sharing them through social media networks. Additionally, you need to be careful sharing information on Facebook, Twitter, and the like about patients you have cared for, ensuring that you do not provide enough detail that the HCO, patient, or staff member could be identified. This same issue applies to electronic (and other) communication throughout the health care delivery system.

Patient Etiquette: How Does This Relate to Patient-Centered Care?

Patient etiquette may seem like a strange topic, but it is relevant to patient-centered care. Kahn (2008) discusses the need for etiquette-based medicine, but this topic seems to get lost in some nursing education programs and experiences. Patients must be treated with respect, but we know that this does not always happen automatically or naturally. Viewing nurses as respectful of patients is also part of the nursing profession's image. Patient etiquette includes items such as asking permission to enter the patient's room and waiting for an answer; introducing yourself, shaking hands, sitting down, and smiling as appropriate; briefly explaining your role on the team; or asking patients how they are feeling and how they feel about their illness and the care they have received. In addition, it is important to ask patients what they want to be called and to provide privacy to patients and families when possible. These actions and attitudes "put professionalism and patient satisfaction at the center of the clinical encounter and bring back some of the elements of ritual that have always been an important part of the healing process" (Kahn 2008, 1988).

Patient Education

Patient education is a complex process and should be included in all nursing curricula. If a patient does not have enough information and quality information, this can affect care and health care decisions. Some areas that require patient education to improve health are identified in the *Quality Chasm* reports, such as tobacco, alcohol, high-fat foods, and firearm injuries (violence). Nurses in public and community health settings typically include such topics in community health education, but patients in other settings also need similar counseling. Patient education must be culturally sensitive because the meanings of health, illness, and death are not the same everywhere.

Keeping the patient in the center of care means that we need to consider what the patient feels is important and listen to them. Patient, family, or community health education should also address safety issues such as prevention of medication errors and its relationship to self-management of care. You must consider health literacy when planning, implementing, and evaluating patient education.

Family or Caregiver Roles: Family-Centered Care

Patient advocacy and PCC are directly related to family-centered care. Family-centered care, like PCC, is a partnership between the family and health care provider. This partnership involves planning and evaluating care with input from the family (which is recognized as important) and expertise and information offered by the health care provider (Seyda, Shelton, and DiVenere 2008). You cannot, however, assume that all patients want their families involved, nor can you take for granted the level of desired family involvement or what information may be shared with the family. Patients must be asked about this before steps are taken to communicate with and include the family. The core principles of family-centered care are dignity and respect, information sharing, participation, and collaboration. As with PCC, the overall goal for family-centered care is better outcomes. Family-centered care has an impact on "improved health outcomes, lower health care costs, more effective allocation of resources, reduced medical errors and litigation, greater patient, family, and professional satisfaction, increased patient/family self-efficacy/advocacy, and improved medical/health education" (Seyda, Shelton, and DiVenere 2008, 66).

Family-centered care may be thought of as relevant only to children's health or pediatric services, but it applies to all patients. The family will likely be involved in the support of a dying patient, such as hospice care; and in caring for older family members, a growing responsibility in the United States. Families can be very important in preventing errors; they have valuable information for health care providers and may observe as care is provided—asking questions, noting differences, and so on. This can lead to fewer errors and improved communication that reduces the likelihood of litigation.

The Patient-Centered Medical Home
Model: A New View of Primary Care

The American Academy of Pediatrics describes the medical home as a model to deliver primary care that is accessible, continuous, comprehensive, family-centered, coordinated, compassionate, and culturally effective (National Center for Medical Home Implementation [NCMHI] 2017). This same model can be applied to adults. The Association of American

Medical Colleges (AAMC) also describes the medical home and proposes that everyone should have access to one (AAMC 2008). In this situation the patient will be able to seek health advice and support through access to consistent, coordinated long-term services. These services should include prevention; care for most problems and is the point of first-contact for that care; coordination of services; integration of care across the health system; and provision of care and health education in a culturally competent manner with consideration of the patient, family, and community (AAMC 2008). The ACA supported the development of methods such as the medical home model (NCMHI 2017).

The medical home model is based on patient-centered care. Individualized care provides preventive care and manages chronic disease, emphasizing collaboration and coordination. Same-day appointments and expanded appointment hours are more available; communication is enhanced through tools like secure e-mail; electronically transmitted prescriptions; and electronic medical or health records (EMRs/EHRs) are used. You can explore and learn more about this concept at the medical home website (https://medicalhomeinfo.aap.org/). What would be the nurse's role, both APRNs and non-APRNs, in this model? Search for more information about medical homes and consider how this new model might affect nursing roles and responsibilities.

Patient- and Family-Centered Rounds

Patient- and family-centered rounds lead to greater patient-centered care (Siserhen et al. 2007). This should be an interprofessional approach, including the patient's family if the patient does not object. Engaging the family is important when the family is a significant part of the patient's life, but in some cases patients may not want family members to hear the information. You should participate in these important learning opportunities. These rounds demonstrate the importance of care that includes the family, interprofessional teams, communication, coordination, and collaboration. It is important to be prepared for these types of rounds—what communication methods are used, what is the general process of rounds, and so on.

Gerontology

The world's population is aging and to provide quality care we need to educate nurses to meet the special needs of older adults. As noted in *Retooling for an Aging America* (IOM 2008), there is a growing need to educate staff so they can effectively care for older adults. There are greater funding opportunities for research and programs to improve this care.

Gerontology should be integrated into all nursing education programs, which should include clinical experiences with this population. Examine this report and its recommendations to improve care for this population.

Clinical Prevention and Population Health: Curricular Framework for Health Professionals

The Essentials of Baccalaureate Education includes "Clinical Prevention and Population Health" as one of its nine essential curricular areas (AACN 2008b). *The Essentials of Doctoral Education* also includes this topic (Maeshiro et al. 2011). The Association for Prevention Teaching and Research (APTR), which collaborates with many federal agencies, offers resources that focus on preventive health care. This website provides modules and other materials to support further understanding of this topic (http://www.aptrweb.org/). There is need for public health leadership that is responsible, uses social strategy and political will, and has interpersonal skills.

The APTR initiative illustrates the impact the *Quality Chasm* reports, in this case the public health reports, have had on health care (see chapter 1). Some of the reports describe the current state of public and community health and the need for changes. Combining them with *Healthy People 2020*, we are again reminded of the importance of the perspectives of populations and the role of all health care professions in health promotion and prevention.

5

Core Competency: Work on Interprofessional Teams

Cooperate, collaborate, communicate, and integrate care in teams to ensure that care is continuous and reliable. (Greiner and Knebel 2003, 4)

Interprofessional teams work collaboratively and collegially, not in parallel. No health professional should plan care in isolation; instead, all team members should work together to plan and implement care.

Teamwork

Marla Salmon has this to say on the topic of teamwork in nursing:

> *I have grown tired of us saying that we are making major strides in collaboration and partnership with others beyond nursing. I worry that we in nursing have fought so hard for our professional identity and autonomy that we see being separate from others as a condition for future success. I see our separateness as antithetical to our most basic professional values. How can we reconcile our commitment to providing the best possible care when we still grapple with the place that nursing assistants, technicians, and others have in relation to our work?* (2007, 117)

Just as Salmon notes, working in interprofessional teams is a difficult competency to accomplish when we continue to keep health care professions separate in most US universities and other educational programs. Health care students are usually socialized for their profession in isolation of other health care professions. This all affects the quality of care. When health care providers do not know how to communicate with one another; when we use abusive language and have conflicts with one another; when we do not understand our different roles and responsibilities and thus do not know how to make the most of what each profession can offer; when we work against each other rather than with each other to provide care; and when we use different terminology, we undermine quality, safe care and are unable to provide patient-centered care (PCC). The National Council of State Boards of Nursing (NCSBN) reported that some of the important factors that relate to nurse involvement in patient errors are ineffective teamwork and limitations in understanding when and how to call the physician (NCSBN 2005; Smith and Crawford 2003).

Interprofessional Collaborative Teams

Precursors to collaboration are individual clinical competence and mutual trust and respect. Collaboration requires shared understanding of goals and roles shared decision-making and effective conflict management. You need to learn how to have a respectful professional dialogue that considers different perspectives. You also need to understand that although the history of nursing has fostered permissive, submissive language and actions, these do not constitute effective professional communication (Gordon 2005).

Care Coordination

Care coordination must be a topic in all courses and clinical experiences from the very beginning of every nursing program, whether undergraduate or graduate (Craig, Eby, and Whittington 2011). What are the roles of the nurse and the roles of other team members? What are the roles of nursing staff and other health care professionals? How can care coordination be improved? What is the integrator role that some nurses play? What can nurses do to improve interprofessional care coordination? How does this role affect adherence to treatment plans and quality of care?

Transformational Leadership

Transformational leadership is highly regarded today, and the *Quality Chasm* reports, for example, *Leadership by Example* and *Keeping Patients*

Safe, consider it the best leadership approach. This, however, does not mean that it is easy to implement—it is not. You need to understand leadership and followership, appreciate how you respond both as a leader and as a follower, and recognize the need to develop your own leadership and followership competencies. What makes an effective leader and an effective follower?

Most health care organizations (HCOs) are in a state of perpetual change. What do you know about the change process? How do you respond to change? You will soon have to step up, take a stand, and be a leader: this should begin while you are a student (for example, serving on a student committee, planning student activities, etc.). The National Student Nurses Association (NSNA) offers information on opportunities for leadership experiences (see http://www.nsna.org).

What is empowerment, and why is it important to nurses? Shared governance is one approach that may develop a productive work climate. When you are in HCOs for clinical experiences, ask questions about leadership and organizational effectiveness within the organization. How does the organization respond to change? How well does the staff trust leadership? Why would this be important to know before taking a new position? Consider why it is important to have a close fit between your personal values and the values and mission of the organization.

Allied Health Team Members

Nursing students need to understand the roles of all possible team members, including allied health members. In 2011 the Health and Medicine Division (HMD) addressed the issue of the growing number of allied health care providers in a workshop. One of the key issues was defining *allied health care providers*:

> *According to Title 42 of the U.S. Code, an allied health professional is a health professional other than a registered nurse or physician assistant who has a certificate, associate's degree, bachelor's degree, master's degree, doctoral degree, or post-baccalaureate training in a science relating to health care and who shares in the responsibility for the delivery of health care services or related services, including: diagnostic, dietary and nutrition, health promotion, rehabilitation, and health care organization or system management.* (Olson 2011)

Search for information about allied health roles and responsibilities and then discuss how the team works together with different types of providers. When you first go into health care settings, identify different team members and observe what they do with patients and their responsibilities as members of the health care team. When you are assigned to work with allied health staff such as licensed practical nurses (LPNs), unlicensed assistive personnel (UAPs), physical therapists (PTs), dieticians, and others, consider their roles and they compare to yours as a nurse.

Student Communication Requirements

Clinical documentation and paperwork seem only to increase and this profusion of paperwork also plagues schools of nursing. Students typically spend much of their time on written assignments. The use of electronic versions of assignments may lead to longer assignments, and we may assume this is more effective learning; however, longer is not necessarily better and nurses need to be concise. It is often difficult for faculty to step back and ask whether the assignments are helpful and aid learning, meet course objectives, or develop competencies. What is the student perspective on the assignments? Requiring nursing students to write everything down may interfere with their ability to think on their feet, discuss an issue or problem, and use critical thinking and clinical reasoning and judgment. Some written assignments accomplish this, but not all. Another example is having students give PowerPoint slide presentations. These presentations can be useful, but we need to offer students experiences in explaining a care problem or sharing an experience with a group without slides as a prop? Using slides does not happen in the real world of daily practice—reports, rounds, and staff meetings. It is always difficult to give up a course activity after it has become routine, but if schools of nursing are to graduate competent entry-level nurses who can function in an ever-changing health care environment, nursing faculty also need to change and be willing to concede that a strategy or learning activity is not yielding the expected outcomes.

Team Communication

Team communication is a critical element in meeting patient needs, providing quality care, and reaching effective patient outcomes. It is critically intertwined with health care professional roles, ability to work with others, recognition that the team is the best method for reaching required goals, and willingness to compromise, collaborate, and coordinate together. It also has a major impact on preventing errors. Structured methods, such as Situation-Background-Assessment-Recommendation (SBAR) and debriefing, are now used by many HCOs to improve team communication.

Written Communication

The team is also an important element of written communication, as teams do not just communicate orally. It is easy for students to view documentation as something done to communicate nurse to nurse; however, there is much more to written communication. It helps the entire health care team communicate the plan of care, what has been done, and outcomes. Not only is documentation important to all the health care providers, but it also provides data for quality improvement (QI) and is essential to reimbursement. There are important legal implications of documentation and written communication, particularly when there are problems. Students must consider all these implications and understand how documentation relates to the five health care professions core competencies.

Verbal Abuse and Incivility

Communication skills are always important and should be developed throughout the curriculum. A growing concern for nurses is verbal abuse from others involved in health care (including other nurses, physicians, and also family members of patients). In fact, verbal abuse is cited as one of the reasons that nursing is such a stressful profession. You need guidance on how to respond and examples of strategies that some HCOs are using to prevent verbal abuse and incivility. Your school of nursing should also support a zero-tolerance policy on verbal abuse or incivility from students, faculty, administrators, or staff, and implement the policy. You need to follow this policy, and after graduation, follow your employer's policy.

Patient-Clinician Communication

Patient-clinician communication is important in health care delivery, particularly quality care. The Joint Commission notes that the most common cause of sentinel events is ineffective communication (TJC 2007). The communication process is closely connected to health care literacy, diversity, and patient education. How do we teach patients? How do we use effective methods to provide patient or family education? Effective patient education has become more difficult because of the fluctuating staff levels; patients who may not be able to concentrate; patient acuity; short lengths of stay; health literacy factors; and the highly stressful health care environment that does not allow much time for staff to even to talk with patients and families.

Staffing, Teams, and Quality: Maximizing Workforce Capability

Keeping Patients Safe: Transforming the Work Environment for Nurses (Child 2004) suggests that staff changes over time (per geographic area, specific HCO, and nationally) and may be a significant risk to patient safety (HRSA 2010). This report describes nurses as the glue that holds HCOs together at the point of care. Nurses serve as integrators to determine patient needs and alert other professionals who are not at the bedside or in the community clinics. In this role, nurses should actively use patient surveillance. If a nurse does not provide surveillance for the health care team, significant patient data may be lost, and often physicians and other professionals may then not be alerted to impending care problems. Some of the work must be delegated to others and some may be transformed by technology; however, this still requires careful consideration based on education and expertise. Many consider this report the tipping point that allows nursing's contribution to patient outcomes to be quantified. This report was completed long before *The Future of Nursing*. It is an important document that recognizes the needs of the staff nurse, the leadership role of the staff nurse and nurse-managers (particularly in relationship to quality care), and reality of the work environment. It is this group of nurses—staff nurses—that provides most of the care and has the greatest impact on the quality of care.

Promoting Safe Staffing Levels: Recruitment and Retention, Implications

Recruitment and retention are related to staffing level and mix, which have an impact on how care is provided and how well it meets standards. When HCOs have problems with staff recruitment and retention this can lead to major care problems. Nursing students need help building job-hunting skills, such as interviewing, looking for a positive work environment, writing résumés and query letters, and matching a job to their competencies and personal needs.

Schools of nursing might also reduce attrition by making it clear to students what they may experience during the first year and cultivating skills such as stress management, assertiveness, and problem solving. Nurse externships and residencies are used by some HCOs to increase recruitment and retention of new graduates, decrease costs related to orientation and turnover, and increase quality of care. You need to understand these options and determine if they would be of benefit to your career plans.

Design of Work Hours and Risks

There is sufficient evidence today to connect staff fatigue with adverse events. Problems with staff fatigue have increased due to longer work hours and have also impacted productivity (TJC 2011). You need information about fatigue and its effects on work, such as slowed reactions, diminished attention to detail, errors of omission, compromised problem-solving, reduced motivation and vigor for successful completion of required tasks, and disrupted circadian rhythms, as well as information on reactions to working a night shift and how shift work is arranged, adjusting to changing hours, and potential impacts on their personal lives. Hughes and Rogers (2004) note that fatigue resulting from insufficient sleep or substandard quality of sleep over an extended period can lead to a number of problems, as noted also by the government and other sources, such as: attention problems, decreased motivation, irritability, problems with memory and confusion, and personal problems such as family conflict, substance abuse, automobile accidents, health problems (psychological and physical), and so on. All of these impact problem-solving, judgment, and reaction time.

Keeping Patients Safe (Child 2004) discusses the need to limit the hours of nurses who provide direct patient care to no more than 12 hours in a 24-hour period and 60 hours in a 7-day period (Child 2004, 13). Several studies indicate that errors increase with increased consecutive hours worked. Rogers and colleagues (2004) note that errors increased threefold when a nurse worked a shift longer than 12.5 hours. Another study of more than six hundred nurses indicates that rotating shifts and inadequate sleep patterns increase the risk of errors (Gold et al. 1992). There have been more studies on this problem, indicating increasing concern about possible negative implications of 12-hour shifts. At the same time, some schools of nursing have moved to using 12-hour shifts for student clinical rotations. This may not be an effective learning schedule, and it also sets up student expectation of this type of scheduling after graduation when some HCOs are trying to move away from it.

Kalisch, Begeny, and Anderson (2008) comment that consistent scheduling is critical to high-level teamwork and does have an impact on errors. They describe the work environment today: an environment with staff moving in and out of a unit based on multiple time schedules. Staff on a single unit may work 3-, 6-, 8-, 10-, and 12-hour shifts. This means that many changes occur in each shift, with multiple staff working different hours. This clearly hampers teams, handoffs, and communication and means that patients must cope with multiple staff members in a 24-hour period. This type of scheduling increases the risk of errors and affects PCC and QI.

The ANA also recognizes that staff fatigue has a major impact on errors and the quality of care and therefore provides a number of resources for nurses on this important topic on its website (2016d). In the past few years, medicine has recognized the impact of fatigue on physician residents and made changes in shifts and hours that reflect the need for sleep during long shifts. Nursing has not done much; in fact, with mandatory overtime, more 12-hour shifts, fluctuating nursing shortages in some areas of the country or in some HCOs, and high patient acuity, nurses are probably more fatigued today than in the past.

It is important to recognize the relationship between staffing, the nursing shortage, leadership, management, HCO administration impact on nursing, quality of care, costs of care, health policies, and regulation such as state board of nursing regulations.

Temporary or Contingent Staff

Health care organizations use temporary or contingent workers (e.g., temporary agency nurses of traveling nurses) to fill empty positions, particularly during shortage periods. This costly solution affects employee morale and quality of care. It is also a growing problem for nursing education as students need supervision and guidance from staff knowledgeable about the HCO. Regular staff must work effectively with temporary staff, helping to orient, support, and integrate them into the work environment.

Delegation

Teamwork is also a critical component of delegation. You need to understand the delegation process and how to apply it. For example, how do surveillance and failure to rescue, topics discussed later, relate to delegation? Delegation identifies what some team members may do on a daily basis in the work setting. It is related to all five health care professions core competencies. To participate in the delegation process, the patient must understand staff roles and responsibilities; patients can then appreciate why certain staff may be providing certain care. There are some aspects of care that patients may be doing for themselves (self-management) or through family members. Quality improvement should be considered during delegation, ensuring that care is provided as needed and is effective, safe, and efficient to meet outcomes. Health information technology (HIT) is applied in team communication and documentation that is done, which are parts of delegation. Evidence-based practice (EBP) and evidence-based management (EBM) provide evidence about what must be done and may also provide evidence about who can best provide which type of care (intervention) to patients. We need much more research to expand available data and evidence, but other important EBP elements (patient values and preferences, assessment data, and clinical expertise) should not be ignored in practice. There is a tendency in discussing EBP to focus only on research evidence, but these other types of evidence need to also be used. The NCSBN website provides a description of the delegation decision tree, delegation and nursing assistive personnel, and other information about delegation (NCSBN 2016a).

Workspace Design and the Work Environment

You probably do not think much about workspace and work environment, but both are important. Assessing a clinical unit can help you to understand the impact of the environment on work and practice; for example, lighting; space; accessibility for patients, families, and staff; nurses' work area; noise level; furnishings; flooring (different flooring can affect fatigue, noise, cleanliness, etc.); traffic through the unit; accessibility of supplies and equipment; space for medication preparation and distractions in that space; documentation system and accessibility; space for private discussion and meetings; access to communication methods (tablets, computer, bulletin boards, etc.); and space for staff to relax. What are the students' first impressions when they step onto the unit? How does the unit atmosphere make them feel? For example, when neonatal intensive care units (NICUs) were open rooms with no noise abatement, most of the nurses felt anxious and tense because of the noise and bright lights. When more attention was paid to dimming lights and banning overhead pages and more units were designed as pods or modules, staff members tended to talk softly, were more mindful of noise and lights, and were less tense.

What is a healing environment, and how can one be created and maintained (Swanson and Wojnar 2004)? How do environment and workspace affect how care is provided and received and how these factors might affect the risk for errors. What could be changed to improve the workspace and work environment? What could be done that is not too costly and complex to make the unit a better place to deliver and receive care?

Training in Teams: Interprofessional Education (IPE)

Interprofessional learning experiences act as a bridge to better professional teamwork and several significant reports have been published recently about interprofessional education (IPE). The World Health Organization, recognizing the importance of interprofessional teams in health care, published an extensive report on interprofessional education, as described in figures in the report (2010). This report was then used as framework for a report on the same topic in the United States (IPEC 2011).

6

Core Competency: Employ Evidence-Based Practice

Integrate best research with clinical expertise and patient values for optimum care, and participate in learning and research activities to the extent feasible. (Greiner and Knebel 2003, 4)

Evidence-based practice (EBP) facilitates the use of research findings in practice; however, there is more than one source of evidence, such as patient values and preferences, history and assessment data, and the health care provider's expertise. The emphasis should be on best evidence, and students need to understand how to select an appropriate level of evidence or evaluate expert opinions and research findings. The tendency is to assume that research is the only type of EBP evidence, when in fact there are several types of evidence. Students may be fearful of research, but they need to embrace a scientific basis for interventions and see the application in practice when provided with sufficient background information about the importance of research findings and their relationship to best practice.

Research

The National Institutes of Health (NIH) Common Fund provided some funding for interdisciplinary research in order to

> *change academic research culture, both in the extramural research community and in the extramural program at the NIH, such that interdisciplinary [interprofessional] approaches are facilitated. The Interdisciplinary Research Program included initiatives to dissolve academic department boundaries within academic institutions and increase cooperation between institutions, train scientists to cultivate interdisciplinary efforts, and build bridges between the biological sciences and the behavioral and social sciences. Collectively, these efforts were intended to change academic research culture so that interdisciplinary [interprofessional] approaches and team science are a normal mode of conducting research and scientists who pursue these approaches are adequately recognized and rewarded.* (NIH 2014)

In 2008, the Robert Wood Johnson Foundation (RWJF) invited proposals for an interprofessional nursing quality research initiative to "generate, disseminate, and translate research on how nurses contribute to and can improve patient care quality" (Naylor et al. 2013). There is a definite trend toward encouraging more interprofessional research, whenever this is applicable.

Nurses need to be involved in research about quality care and participate in evaluating how nursing care is connected to quality care. The reports recommend expanding nursing research to increase the nursing profession's understanding of the relationship between quality care and nursing, outcomes, and the role of nurses and interprofessional collaborations.

In addition to curriculum changes, funding streams for health care organizations (HCOs) are also influenced by the Health and Medicine Division (HMD). As noted in the *Quality Chasm* reports, the Agency for Healthcare Research and Quality (AHRQ) should fund research to evaluate how the current regulatory and legal systems facilitate or inhibit the changes needed for the twenty-first-century health care delivery system, and how they can be modified to support health care professionals and HCOs working to accomplish the six aims of care: safe, timely, effective, efficient, equitable, and patient-centered (STEEEP; IOM 2001). This work has yet to be completed. Nursing should be involved so that nursing input can be included; issues critical to nursing, such as licensure and liability, are involved in this recommendation. The multiple-state compact on licensure, which has been instituted in some states, is one example of thinking outside the box.

Nursing education is involved in research. Some schools of nursing are studying quality issues, though more should, as nursing is directly involved in quality of care. One area that requires further exploration is how education affects student performance and future performance in the workplace. Examples of other potential areas for nursing research related to quality are:

- Fragmentation of care
- Errors and error prevention
- Surveillance
- Safe medication administration
- Application of National Healthcare Quality and Disparities Report (QDR) results
- Nursing leadership
- Impact of medical and information technology
- Implementation of the five health care professions core competencies in the curriculum and in practice
- Centers for Medicare and Medicaid Services (CMS) initiatives focused on prevention of hospital-acquired conditions, such as patient falls, and reduction in thirty-day unplanned readmissions
- Care coordination
- Teamwork (including its impact on care and its implementation in education)
- Operating room and surgical procedures to reduce errors
- Emergency department practices and procedures
- Management of diagnostic tests, screening, and information
- Intensive care units: adult, neonatal, pediatric
- Care of frail elderly (for example, medication safety, coordination of care, falls, and decubiti)
- Quality improvement (QI) and making changes in practice
- Effective use of QI methods such as Plan, Do, Study, Act (PDSA), failure modes and effects analysis (FMEA), checklists, and methods to reduce workarounds and improve handoffs

Evidence-Based Practice

Sigma Theta Tau defines *evidence-based practice* as the "integration of best clinical practice, research evidence, nursing expertise, and the values and preferences of the individuals, families, and communities who are served" (2006, 3).

When possible, care intervention choices should be supported with evidence such as clinical guidelines available from the National Guideline Clearinghouse (https://www.guideline.gov/). Systematic reviews offer examinations of multiple primary investigations addressing a particular question, practice guidelines, and how to use computer-based clinical decision support systems. Evidence-based clinical guidelines promote quality of care and should be incorporated in all courses. For example, you can review guidelines and consider how the guidelines might affect the care for a specific health problem and population. The AHRQ evidence-based practice centers are important resources for students and nursing staff. The nursing profession should be actively involved in the development of EBP centers and application of the EBP process, and then ensure that nurses can access information relevant to nursing care. You may also use the Joanna Briggs Institute and Cochrane reviews as resources for EBP.

EBP must to be embedded in nursing care, but to accomplish this it must be embedded in nursing education. This also applies to continuing education (CE). The NAS/HMD and others recommend that health care CE move to an interprofessional education approach, including physicians, nurses, pharmacists, and so on, and when applicable CE should be based on EBP (IOM 2010c; Davies et al. 2003). This approach would support all of the health care professions core competencies.

Collaborative Evidence-Based Practice

Nursing is focusing on the application of EBP specific to nursing, and other health care professions are focusing on their own EBP. Certainly each profession has to do this; however, health care professions must also work collaboratively in their EBP efforts. With the increased need to use inter-professional teams, each specific team needs to consider interprofessional aspects of EBP for patient care—all aspects of care, keeping the patient in the center of EBP, and all elements of EBP (research, clinician expertise, patient preferences and values, and patient history and assessment data). In addition, QI covers all areas of care, and use of EBP should improve care, again requiring a collaborative effort. When patients are divided into domains or territories by different health care professions, it is not possible to provide PCC: the risk of errors increases and quality of care declines. Doctor Robin Newhouse comments, "Despite the clear need to work together for a common patient-centered approach, professions tend to approach improvements in care by setting boundaries around their scope-specific activities. Profession-specific patient goals are important, but must also be integrated into unified action" (2008, 416).

Patient engagement and PCC are central to interprofessional collaborative practice, which includes EBP. A new agency has been formed, mandated by the ACA of 2010, called the Patient-Centered Outcomes Research Institute (PCORI). It is designed to fund research focusing on the production of evidence-based information (http://www.pcori.org/). This agency is linked with AHRQ in an effort to ensure that evidence-based guidelines are used and adapted for the patient population so that the patient and family understand the treatment plan. The PCORI website provides information that can be used in teaching.

Evidence-Based Management

There should be greater emphasis on evidence-based management (EBM; Pfeffer and Sutton 2006; Marshall 2008):

> *Reports of medical mistakes have splashed across newspapers and magazines in the United States. At the same time, instances of overuse, underuse, and misuse of management tactics and strategies receive far less attention. The sense of urgency associated with improving the quality of medical care does not exist with respect to improving the quality of management decisions. Taking a more evidence-based approach would improve the competence of the decision-makers and their motivation to use more scientific methods when making a decision.* (Kovner and Rundall 2009, 53)

One of the American Organization of Nurse Executives (AONE) strategic objectives is greater use of EBM (AONE 2012). You need to understand EBM, which applies best evidence to management decisions to improve decisions and performance (Kovner and Rundall 2009). The EBM process is similar to the EBP process: identify a question, search for evidence, assess the quality of that evidence, apply the best evidence, and evaluate outcomes. As is true with EBP, but even more so with EBM, it is not always easy to find management research to use as evidence in decision-making.

7

Core Competency:
Apply Quality Improvement

*Identify errors and hazards in care; understand
and implement basic safety design principles,
such as standardization and simplification;
continually understand and measure quality of
care in terms of structure, process, and outcomes
in relation to patient and community needs;
and design and test interventions to change
processes and systems of care, with the objective of
improving quality.* (Greiner and Knebel 2003, 4)

This core competency has come to the forefront due to the ongoing concerns for patient safety and the role of medication errors.

The *Quality Chasm* findings on patient safety and error rates have made quality improvement (QI) a vital concern and expanded the need to focus on quality of care in general, not just errors. Nurses need to be prepared to participate actively in the QI process, serving as leaders when needed. Many of the *Quality Chasm* reports have existed now for many years. We are improving today, but at a very slow rate. The National Healthcare Quality and Disparities Report (QDR), administered by the Agency for Healthcare Research and Quality (AHRQ), provides us with an annual report; however, the most current report is always a year behind the current date.

Developing a Health Care Quality Framework: Definition of Quality

Quality is not easy to define. The traditional view of quality is shown in figure 7-1.

Donabedian's quality model describes each of the major components (1980):

- **Structure:** System characteristics, provider characteristics, and patient characteristics, or the environment in which care is provided
- **Process:** Technical style and interpersonal style, or the manner in which care is provided
- **Outcomes:** Clinical end points or results, satisfaction with care, functional status of the patient

Discussing quality related to each of these components and how they interact allows you to gain a perspective on the dynamic quality process. The Institute of Medicine (IOM) supports these components and defines *quality care* as "the degree to which health services for individuals and populations increase the likelihood of desired health outcomes and are consistent with current professional knowledge (Lohr 1990, as cited in Institute of Medicine 2001, 432).

We need more content about QI for students in all health care professions and more application of this content. If this is done effectively, students will enter their respective professions with greater knowledge of QI, motivated to improve care with the ability to participate actively in the QI process. The following domains of core content for QI continue to apply: recognition that health care is a process with variation and needs to be measured; importance of the customer, including patient preferences as noted in the patient-centered care (PCC) model; recognition of change as a critical component of the health care system; effective collaboration and accountability; recognition of the need to understand social context related to health and care delivery; and application of knowledge (Batalden 1998).

Critical Quality Definitions: Reducing Errors and Improving Safety

The *Quality Chasm* reports expand knowledge about safety and errors as part of their examination of quality care, including definitions of key terms. Common terminology facilitates communication among health care professions and improves data collection and analysis. The following terms and examples are relevant to nurses involved in initiatives to reduce

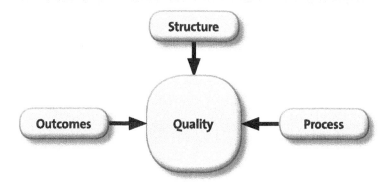

FIGURE 7-1. **The elements of quality**

errors and improve safety (Kohn, Corrigan, and Donaldson 1999; Chassin and Galvin 1998):

- **Safety:** Freedom from accidental injury.

  Example: The patient leaves the hospital after surgery and a three-day stay with expected outcomes reached and no complications or errors.

- **Error:** The failure of a planned action to be completed as intended or the use of an inadequate plan to achieve an aim. Errors are directly related to outcomes and harm the patient.

  Example: The patient is given the wrong medication (error of execution).

- **Adverse event:** An injury resulting from a medical intervention, not due to the patient's underlying condition. Not all adverse events are due to errors and not all are preventable. Error analysis is needed to determine the relationship of an error to an adverse event.

  Example: The patient is given the wrong medication and experiences a seizure. If the patient does not have a seizure disorder, this is most likely a preventable adverse event, but more must be discovered about the causes. Would this medication error normally cause a seizure? Are there other possible causes for the seizure? How did the error happen that led to the adverse event?

- **Misuse:** Avoidable complications that prevent patients from receiving full potential benefit of a service.

  Example: The patient receives a medication that is not prescribed and conflicts with the patient's allergies; the patient experiences anaphylaxis.

- **Overuse:** Potential for harm that exceeds the possible benefit from a service.

  Example: An older patient is taking multiple medications, some of which may interact negatively, and the patient's multiple health care providers are not aware of the medications prescribed by different specialists.

- **Underuse:** Failure to provide a service that would have produced a favorable outcome for the patient.

  Example: The patient is not able to get specialty treatment needed for cancer because of distance from health care services, or the patient's insurer will not reimburse for an arthritis medication that could make the patient more mobile.

- **Near miss:** Recognition that an event occurred that *might* have led to an adverse event. This means the error almost happened. It is important to understand such errors; they provide valuable information for preventing future actual errors.

  Example: The surgical team is preparing for knee surgery. The right knee is prepped, but when a team member checks the records, the team member finds out that it is the left knee that requires surgery. An error was prevented, but why was the wrong knee initially prepped?

- **Active error:** An error that results from noncompliance with a procedure (Reason 1990).

  Example: A nurse does not check vital signs required to confirm the need for a specific medication. The medication is administered when the patient does not need it, and the patient experiences negative side effects.

- **Latent conditions:** Threats not immediately apparent. These indicate problems in the system (Reason 1990).

  Example: Some staff members are not familiar with a change in policy, though it is assumed that all are implementing the new policy. An error occurs due to lack of knowledge of the change.

- **Sentinel event:** An event that has a drastic negative outcome; unexpected death, serious physical or psychological injury, or serious risk. A root cause analysis of the event is conducted to examine the process. The goal is not to place blame but to prevent future events.

  Example: The patient commits suicide while in the hospital for treatment.

- **Root cause analysis:** In-depth analysis of an error to assess the event and identify causes and possible solutions that includes representatives from critical staff groups. Root cause analysis uses multiple methods to collect and analyze data related to an error and determine best solutions or responses.

The World Health Organization identifies common causes of adverse events and types of adverse events on its website (WHO 2008). This information is useful for development of simulations, scenarios, cases, and other learning activities for students.

Simple Rules for QI in the Twenty-First Century

Crossing the Quality Chasm identifies simple rules that should be considered as care is improved (Table 3-1, IOM 2001, 67). Even though these rules were first described in 2001, this report compares approaches (old rules) with new rules for health care delivery, providing a vision for US health care that still applies. The rules represent the philosophical direction or vision recommended for the health care system. Consider how your own professional experiences relate to these rules:

- Compare the current rule with the new rule.
- How does each rule apply to nursing practice? What changes are needed to meet each new rule?
- How does each rule affect interprofessional teamwork?

Entering students can be asked to discuss their perspectives on the rules—their personal view of health care—and then to reflect on them again at the end of the nursing program. Your perspectives should change over the course of your education. You will understand these new rules and be prepared to use them in your nursing practice.

Six Aims: STEEEP

Crossing the Quality Chasm identifies six major quality improvement aims that should be considered and adopted by all health care providers, including nurses. Reviewing these aims, one might wonder, "Aren't we doing this already?" Perhaps, but we are not doing it routinely or effectively. On one level, these aims are not surprising; they might seem obvious and straightforward to the point of being overly simplistic. However, these aims, often referred to as STEEP, are not as intuitive as they may seem. Though imperative, they are not consistently applied. All six of these elements are related to nursing practice (IOM 2001, 42–53):

1. **Safe.** Avoiding injuries that harm patients from the care that is intended to help them. *How does this apply to your patient care?*

2. **Timely.** Reducing waits and possible harmful delays for both patients who receive care and those who give care. Problems with timeliness can lead to physical harm, and even more frequently cause emotional stress. Such problems also affect the patient's trust in the system. *How does time affect your patient care delivery and quality?*

3. **Efficient.** Avoiding waste, including waste of equipment, supplies, ideas, and energy. Better use of resources reduces costs and makes resources more available to those who need them. *How often do you consider efficiency when providing patient care?*

4. **Effective.** Providing services based on scientific knowledge to all who could benefit, and refraining from providing services to those who are not likely to benefit (avoiding underuse and overuse). Effective care implies evidence-based health care with integration of best evidence, clinical expertise, and patient values (Sackett, Rosenberg, and Gray 1996). *How does this apply to patient care you provide?*

5. **Equitable.** Providing care that does not vary in quality because of personal characteristics such as gender, ethnicity, geographic location, and socioeconomic status. Access to care and health care disparities have become major concerns in the United States. There is increased emphasis on diversity training, but it is not yet clear whether this training improves the situation or which type of approach is the best to take. *How does this apply to patient care you provide?*

6. **Patient-centered.** Provide care that is respectful of and responsive to individual patient preferences, needs, and values. The key focus is on the patient's experience of illness and health care. It is quite clear that patients are entering the health care system more informed than in the past due to the increased accessibility of health information. Patients need support in their efforts to be more informed, and nurses have long been advocates of patients and patient education. However, many nurses have little time to educate patients or guide them to needed information. This problem must be resolved from both the nursing education and practice perspectives. How are students taught about patient education? Are they provided with education interventions that are easy to apply, or are these proposed interventions unrealistic given the nature of the work environment today? Most schools of nursing would say that patient education is included in their curricula. However, many probably have not reviewed their content and teaching approaches based on the following: Are the patient education methods used today effective given the current health care environment (rapid turnover of patients, acuity of patients, staff shortages, and work issues)? Are we making the best use of technology in patient education? *How you are providing patient-centered care?*

Each of the aims is highly relevant to nursing and has implications for nurse managers and health care organizations (HCOs). What examples have you observed in HCOs? How do each of the aims affect patients as the aims are integrated into the plan of care? How do the aims affect an aggregate or population? What can be done to resolve problems that may block meeting these aims? The aims may conflict at times, and it is important for you to know how this may occur and how such conflicts can be resolved. For example, can safe care always be efficient? Some of this discussion will involve ethical and legal issues and should integrate standards and the code of ethics (American Nurses Association [ANA] 2015a, 2015c).

Data Collection and Analysis

Data collection and analysis are critical now in health care. Assessment of the three elements of quality care (structure, process, outcomes) requires data that meet regulation requirements, can be used to determine performance, can be applied to accreditation or recognition requirements (e.g., The Joint Commission, Magnet Recognition Program) and in the QI process, and can be used for research (Glassman and Rosenfeld 2015)

Data are also part of documentation. Health information technology (HIT) is used now in all areas of health care from clinics to administration and is also a critical component of QI, not only as a method for improving care but also as a provider of data to determine performance. Examples of HIT methods to improve care are bar coding and decision support systems. Examples of HIT providing data to improve care and HCO functions are health care financial data, risk management and utilization management data, and HCO planning and related data. Access to data has grown so much in health care that it is now referred to as "Big Data." This large amount of data requires that we use methods to organize it in databases (Glassman and Rosenfeld 2015). You need to understand data and the application of data both for improving care and for using in the QI measurement process. Nurses should be and are involved in collecting, analyzing, and arriving at decisions to respond to the problems described by data.

A major problem with data today is information overload. We experience it in our personal lives and professional lives. HCOs are already inundated with information and the greater emphasis placed on QI and EBP has increased the drive for more data. *Information* or *cognitive overload* is defined as "an interpretation that people in response to breakdowns, interruptions of ongoing projects, or imbalances between demand and capacity" (Weick 2009, 76). What influences overload? Examples are interruptions; time pressures; greater demands on cognitive capacity created by more task demands or more complex tasks; attentional factors like decreased scanning or memory problems; stressors (personal and work-related); and the work environment (Sitterding 2015). We need better understanding of the invisible work of nursing to help nurses prevent information overload problems and respond effectively. The Cognitive Work of Nursing Framework, described in figure 7-2, focuses on the relationships between the following factors (Sitterding and Ebright 2015, 13):

- Environmental factors (Work Complexity Contributors)
- Cognitive work leading to decisions about care (Clinical Reasoning-in-Transition)
- Immediate outcomes of the cognitive work (Clinical Judgment)
- Nursing care delivered and patient, nurse, and system outcomes

Patient and Family Roles in Improving Care

Moving beyond having consumers (patients, families) participate in health care decision-making, the newest issue in patient-centered health care is the importance of consumers' role in preventing errors. You do not have to be a health care provider to participate in error prevention. The airline industry actively involves travelers in error prevention; for example, preparing for takeoff and landing and stowing baggage safely to prevent injuries. Why not do the same in health care?

Patient-centeredness emphasizes the patient's role, the partnership between the patient and health care providers, and patient empowerment. Safety improvement should be part of this partnership. Health care professionals need to recognize that they are not the only persons involved in health care delivery and quality. If safety is a system property, then the entire health care system should be designed to prevent errors. This would include everyone involved—all staff, professional and nonprofessional, and patients and families. Different people may observe different safety issues, enhancing the ability to catch errors before they lead to problems. We need transparent health care processes, accessible to all who need or want to know about them (Spath 2008).

What are some examples of situations in which patients should give feedback to prevent errors? Patients and families can easily identify many issues, such as problems with universal precautions, handwashing, medications, cleanliness, slips and falls, clutter, and even medication administration (Spath 2008). In some hospitals, patients and families are encouraged

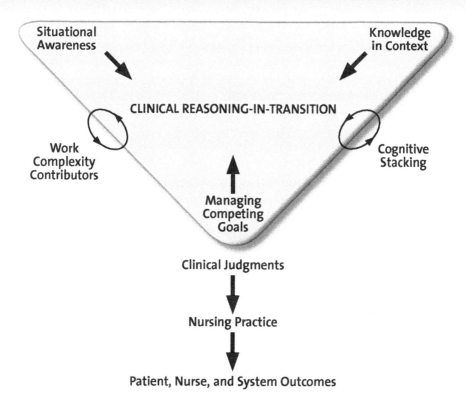

FIGURE 7-2. **Cognitive Work of Nursing Framework overview**
Source: Sitterding, M., and P. Ebright. 2015. "Information Overload: A Framework for Explaining the Issues and Creating Solutions." In *Information Overload: Framework, Tips, and Tools to Manage in Complex Healthcare Environments*, edited by M. Sitterding and M. Broome, 11–33. Silver Spring, MD: American Nurses Association.

to call rapid response teams if they feel the need for special assistance and are not getting responses from staff. Broader areas that would benefit from patient involvement include reaching an accurate diagnosis; deciding best treatment; choosing an experienced, safe provider with current, appropriate certification and verified training; ensuring that treatment is appropriately administered, monitored, and followed; and quickly identifying side effects or adverse events and taking appropriate action in a timely manner (Vincent and Coulter 2002).

Culture of Safety in the Health Care Organization
Moving away from a blame culture to a culture of safety in which everyone serves as a safety inspector is new for health care. It is easier to blame an

individual for an error, as HCOs have done for a long time. However, most errors are due to system, not human, failures. We need to move away from a punitive environment and focus more on learning environments that foster communication about errors and improvement. This is also known as a "no-blame culture" or a "just culture."

HCOs are now focusing on instituting a just culture or culture of safety approach to errors, deemphasizing blame (Boysen 2013; Nurse.com 2008; Dekker 2007). This is a nonpunitive, fair, and just system, though there still must be personal and professional accountability for one's practice actions. Health care professionals must also be accountable for QI activities (Nurse.com 2008). This environment is one in which managers are engaged in the QI processes and in QI and talk routinely and openly with staff about QI issues such as risks and results. All staff are expected to use methods to ensure early recognition of safety risks. The reporting of incidents is seen as an opportunity to identify and respond to QI problems. Human errors may require changes in processes, design, policies and procedures, work environment, or education and training. Interventions to reduce at-risk behaviors include removing incentives for at-risk behaviors, creating incentives for healthy behaviors, and increasing situational awareness to recognize risk factors.

Some clinical areas are more prone to errors due to the nature of the care and environment, such as intensive care units (ICUs) and emergency departments (EDs). These environments require speed in decision-making and action, which increases the risk for errors (Gaskill 2008). This calls for greater efforts to prevent errors, but accepting that errors will not always be prevented is important in establishing a just culture. It takes time to develop and maintain a cultural transformation that rewards instead of penalizes staff for reporting errors and near misses. Staff need to feel safe mentioning near misses and errors and then become part of the solution. Administration needs to recognize that increased reporting of errors and near misses is not a bad sign; *not* reporting is much more serious. When you are in high-risk clinical areas, you need to be more alert for errors. What are examples of high-risk activities and ways in which errors during these activities might be prevented?

What happens when an error occurs and a student and faculty are involved? How comfortable do faculty and students feel about reporting a near miss or an error (disclosure)? Is there a process at the school, similar to the process in the clinical setting, for analyzing errors so students can learn from it, or are errors swept under the rug, with little opportunity for students and faculty to discuss and express their own reactions to making errors? If we do the latter, we are teaching students that this type of response is acceptable in practice after graduation. It is not. Schools of nursing need an error policy and procedure, and this topic needs to be discussed with students. When errors occur and must be disclosed to patients, staff need to carefully consider how this will be done. Many HCOs now are developing policies and procedures that consider issues such as describing the mistake, beliefs about the mistake, staff emotions before and after the mistake, how to cope with the mistake, and how to develop and implement the necessary changes (Banja 2005).

When students or faculty make an error and disclosure is necessary, what communication factors should be considered? These are the same factors and processes that staff need to consider and clarify before talking with the patient (Banja 2005). The patient's physician should speak with the patient, and attorneys should not be present, unless the patient insists on this. In the past, HCO or individual health care provider attorneys might be present but this is no longer recommended. Recording the meeting with the patient should not be done unless the patient wants a recording. It is important to carefully select the location for the conversation with the patient; for example, consider privacy, noise level, potential for interruptions, and so on. There is no doubt that a malpractice lawsuit is a risk. In the discussion, all involved should realize the importance of the communication process—talking directly to the patient, sitting and showing empathy, giving time for the patient to respond and ask questions, and not overdoing what is said. It is okay to apologize but blame should not be part of the conversation.

In order to create and sustain a culture of safety, the process must include (1) an understanding of the essential elements, (2) an understanding of the barriers to creating the culture, (3) strategies for creating the culture, and (4) an evaluation of the results or outcomes (Child 2004). Safety orientation is necessary to prepare staff and maintain knowledge of safety. Trust is crucial when staff members are asked to report errors and near misses: What will be the reaction, and will staff be blamed? Nurses face a major hurdle in accepting this new safety culture because "nurses are trained to believe that clinical perfection is an attainable goal" (Child 2004, 298) and that "'good' nurses do not make errors" (Banister, Butt, and Hackel 1996, as cited in Child 2004, 298). Every nursing program should examine its culture periodically and dispel such unrealistic expectations, providing an atmosphere for open discussion.

Root Cause Analysis

Currently, root cause analysis is used by most hospitals and many other HCOs to analyze errors. This method supports the view that errors typically have system causes that must be understood to improve care. You need to know about this method, as you will be involved in it when you take nursing positions. You also need to practice using it (for example, in simulations). The root cause analysis steps are:

- What happened (described in detail)?
- Who was involved?
- When did it happen?
- Where did it happen?
- What is the severity of the actual or potential harm?
- What is the chance it will happen again?
- What are the consequences?

An interprofessional team representing key stakeholders should do this analysis. At the end of the process, the team should be able to identify prevention strategies. There are resources on the Internet that can assist you in understanding this topic, such as the AHRQ, The Joint Commission, and the Institute for Health Improvement (IHI).

Analyze Errors: A Student Experience

In developing an environment of learning rather than blame and avoiding the blame game, staff and students need to learn from near-miss and error experiences. Policies and standards must be clear. Communication must be open. What do you think will happen if you report a near miss or an error? Do you know the difference between the two? What is your attitude toward errors? What do you see happening related to safety in the HCOs where you go for clinical experience?

It is important to understand the implications of human factors that may be related to the errors, but human factors are not always the cause. Analyze the event, causes, circumstances, conditions, associated procedures, and devices that may be involved. You need to understand this process well enough to use it in your own clinical practice. What are the effects of stressors such as fatigue, interruptions, noise, job dissatisfaction, communication and incivility, burnout, work overload, shift work, family issues, and organizational politics on error rates? Include specific examples of legal issues, standards of practice, nurse practice acts, and documentation of errors so that you are aware of the connection between safety and errors and legal and regulatory issues. The ANA *Code of Ethics for Nurses* and nursing standards are related to your analysis of errors (ANA 2015b; 2015a).

Errors and Related Issues

As mentioned earlier, the report on patient safety defines *safety* as "freedom from accidental injury" (Kohn, Corrigan, and Donaldson 1999, 18) and an *error* as "the failure of a planned action to be completed as intended (error of execution) or the use of a wrong plan to achieve an aim (error of planning)" (Reason 1990, as cited in Kohn, Corrigan, and Donaldson 1999, 28). Though the report defines error, there is no health care consensus on the definition, and there have been disagreements about what actually constitutes an error. For example, some physicians do not consider the following to be errors: delays in treatment, use of outmoded treatment, failure to use needed diagnostic tests, failure to act on test results, mistakes in administration of treatment, and failure to communicate practice variances, suboptimal outcomes, and differences in clinical judgment. In some situations, nurses also agree that these examples are not errors (Mason 2004). Progress has been made in raising awareness about errors, developing reporting systems, and establishing national data collection standards.

Some error-reduction strategies continue to be important even over a long period of time, even more important than in the past, and should be considered when designing learning activities related to QI (Leape 1994; Leape et al. 1991):

- **Reduce reliance on memory.** Use checklists, computerized decision forms, and protocols.
- **Improve information access.** Use informatics placed as close to the point of care as possible; for example, tablets, smartphones, computers on rolling carts, and so on.
- **Make processes as error-proof as possible.** Use prevention methods such as computer safeguards that send up "red flags" to alert for error; for example, allergy alerts as one inputs orders, alerts to fall risk as one documents, and so on.
- **Standardize tasks.** Ensure tasks are done in a consistent manner. This requires clear communication and updating when necessary.
- **Reduce the number of handoffs.** Decrease handoffs and improve the handoff process when it must be used; for example, use a standardized communication method to ensure critical information is always shared.

Risk for Errors

The AHRQ (2003) identified the following as factors that may increase the risk for errors:

- Communication problems, verbal and written, among all types of health care providers
- Inadequate information flow throughout the continuum of care
- Patient-related issues, such as lack of patient education and health literacy problems
- Poor organizational knowledge transfer, such as lack of appropriate orientation and staff education
- Inadequate staffing patterns, such as inadequate staffing, lack of appropriate supervision in situations that are at high risk for errors, and inappropriate staff mix and preparation
- Technical failures, such as medical equipment not functioning, staff unfamiliar with equipment, poor maintenance of equipment, and computer problems limiting access
- Inadequate policies and procedures

Near Misses and Students

When near misses occur, consider the type of near-miss error. How did you recognize the near miss? What are your reactions to and feelings on near misses? What steps could you have taken to prevent the error? Using root cause analysis, look at system processes and consider factors that contributed to the near miss. If an error occurred, this same process can be used to learn more about the error. It is easy to jump to the conclusion that the problem was insufficient staff, but you need to consider other possible causes for the near miss (or error, if one occurred), and then identify possible interventions.

In one study, Dickson and Flynn (2012) examine how staff nurses use clinical reasoning to prevent errors. You need to use clinical reasoning to ensure medication safety by using, for example, these safety practices: educating patients, taking everything into consideration, advocating for patients with pharmacy, coordinating care with physicians, conducting independent medication reconciliation, and verifying with colleagues (Dickson and Flynn 2012). Clinical reasoning is also part of understanding nurse responses in the work environment, particularly as they relate to medication administration. Four factors are important: (1) coping with interruptions and distractions, (2) interpreting physician orders, (3) documenting 'near misses,' (4) and encouraging open communication among team members. The investigators use the following definition of clinical reasoning for their study: "Clinical reasoning in nursing is a complex cognitive process that uses formal and informal thinking strategies to gather and analyze patient information, evaluate the significance of this information and weigh alternative actions" (Dickson and Flynn 2012, 1155; Simmons 2010). We need to examine more thoroughly how clinical reasoning affects a variety of nursing interventions and how it can be used to improve care. The information from this study is highly relevant to nursing education.

Omissions or Missed Nursing Care

Missed nursing care has gained more attention as HCOs give more attention to QI. What is missed nursing care? It is "any aspect of standard, required nursing care this is not provided—errors of omission" (Kalisch 2015, 17). Figure 7-3 describes a model of missed nursing care that integrates structure, process, and outcomes. As illustrated in this model, missed nursing care or omissions impact both staff and patient outcomes in multiple ways. Examples of missed nursing care are not ambulating or

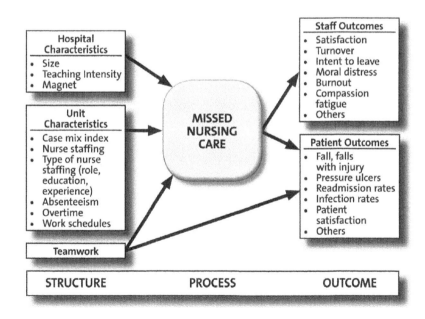

FIGURE 7-3. **Missed Nursing Care Model**
    Source: Kalisch, B. 2015. *Errors of Omission: How Missed Nursing Care Imperils Patients*. Silver Spring, MD: American Nurses Association, 13.

turning a patient every two hours; not assessing the effectiveness of medications; neglecting patient education; not responding to a call light within the expected time; not monitoring intake and output; and not providing adequate mouth care (Kalisch 2015).

Nursing is more than what we do, but we must be alert for what does not get done, which is an error with possible consequences. What factors might increase the risk for missed nursing care? How might this information be used to prevent these errors, for example, inadequate staffing, teamwork problems, poor communication, inadequate patient planning, unexpected increase in workload, inaccessibility of equipment and supplies when needed, unclear policies and procedures, and poor planning? Kalisch reviewed many studies on missed nursing care and concludes that it is "extensive and widespread" (2015, 33).

Medications and Administration: Errors

An intervention with a high risk of errors is medication administration, particularly given the increasing number of drugs, unfamiliar drugs, inadequate math proficiency, environmental stresses (e.g., interruptions, fatigue, overwork, and miscommunication), illegible orders, lack of patient information, and problems with equipment. Bar codes, unit dose dispensing, smart infusion pumps, reference resources, and drug training can all reduce errors. Administering medications safely is one of the critical competencies that any nursing student learns.

The National Coordinating Council for Medication Error Reporting and Prevention (NCC MERP) believes that the quality of data is more important than the number of errors; in other words, there should be no acceptable incidence rates for medication errors (Gallagher and Nadzam 2015; NCC MERP 2002). Given this viewpoint, HCOs should continually improve systems that prevent harm to patients due to medication errors. Monitoring actual and potential medication errors and root cause analysis of errors should not stop, and there should be efforts to identify strategies to reduce these errors.

A study by Harding and Petrick (2008) examines medication errors made and reported by nursing students. This retrospective review identifies three categories of errors that can serve as a guide in reducing errors.

- **Rights violations.** Does the rights-of-administration approach that we are taught to use and teach students lead to narrow thinking because the rights do not consider the system context? Do we isolate our teaching too much by separating patient rights, system parts, and knowledge so that students do not know how to synthesize all of this information?

- **System factors.** The full context of the work setting in which medication is administered may contribute to errors. Often errors in this category have something to do with the medical administration record (MAR), but there is much more to it. System factors include the room where medications are prepared: Are there issues with privacy, noise, and interruptions? Are there problems with the pharmacy processes and how the pharmacy interacts with the unit and nurses? Are problems inherent throughout the entire medication administration process? Problem- and simulation-based strategies improve students' understanding of work-environment issues.

- **Knowledge and understanding.** Gaps in knowledge or understanding can and do lead to errors.

The Joint Commission and the Food and Drug Administration (FDA) publish medications and medication administration alerts on their websites.

Medication administration is a multiphase process (prescribing, transcribing, dispensing, administering, and monitoring), and each phase has the potential for errors (Harding and Petrick 2008; Wolf 2001). The highest rates of error occur in the ordering phase (49–56 percent of the errors), and the second highest is the administration phase (26–40 percent) (Manno 2006; Ackroyd-Stolarz, Hartnell, and MacKinnon 2005). Wolf (2001) identifies nine steps in the typical cycle of medication administration. Students report that distractions during administration led to many of their errors. According to studies by Hughes and Ortiz (2005) and Manno (2006), 27 percent of the errors are due to distraction, so students need to learn how to cope with distractions. Some of this can be incorporated in simulation experiences. Errors of omission are high, at 34 percent (Manno 2006; Hughes and Ortiz, 2005). The common element in many of these errors is the MAR; for example, lack of experience in reading or interpreting the MAR.

With more patients taking more prescription, over-the-counter, and complementary medications and substances, errors have increased. You need to know about all the medication administration steps, issues with multiple drug use, patient and caregiver education, how to question conflicting orders, and how to assess patient medications. Simulation scenarios that include multiple drug orders assist students in identifying appropriate orders, drug interactions, dosages, and administration. What do you think are the typical medication errors based on an analysis of the medication procedure? What corrective actions would you take and what might prevent future errors?

Medication Reconciliation

Medication reconciliation is "the process of avoiding such inadvertent inconsistencies across transitions of care by reviewing the patient's complete medication regimen at the time of admission, transfer, and discharge and comparing it with the regimen being considered for the new setting of care" (Patient Safety Network [PSNet] 2015b). The medication reconciliation process can decrease medication errors and patient harm. To accomplish this, HCOs need policies and procedures that assign primary responsibility for the task, identify time frames for completion, use standardized forms that are easily accessible and visible at all times during the transfer, and clarify all medication discrepancies with the prescribing physician (Resar and Midelfort 2008; Ketchum, Grass, and Padwojski 2005). How is this relevant for students? They need to know about medication reconciliation, appreciate its importance, and understand and apply the process. This can be discussed during content on medication administration and applied in simulation and during clinical experiences; for example, in a home care experience students can review all the medications the patient is taking.

The AHRQ has developed a tool kit, *Medications at Transitions and Clinical Handoffs (MATCH) Toolkit for Medication Reconciliation* (Gleason et al. 2011). The toolkit content notes that medication reconciliation is a complex process that affects all patients as they move through health care settings. This comparison of the patient's current medication regimen against physician orders is done to identify discrepancies. Any discrepancies noted are discussed with the prescriber, and the order is modified, if necessary. Although this toolkit is based on processes developed in acute care settings, the core processes, tools, and resources can be adapted for use in post-acute facilities. PSNet also provides additional information about medication errors in general (PSNet 2015a).

Failure to Rescue

Hospitals are particularly concerned about this issue today, though it can arise in any patient setting. The "intent of the failure to rescue indicator is to measure the hospital's ability to rescue patients that have developed a serious complication" (Manojlovich and Talsma 2007, 504). The AHRQ and the National Quality Forum (NQF) have described this indicator as a critical performance measure; however, there is no consensus on its definition, which limits the ability to collect this data from one health care organization to another.

Two important nursing activities that can prevent FTR are surveillance and taking action when a life-threatening patient complication develops (Clarke and Aiken 2003). There are multiple possible common causes of failure to rescue, such as inadequate monitoring (surveillance); failure to recognize data that implies increased risk for the patient; failure of the HCO to provide clear criteria as to when to take action; failure to complete required monitoring; increased risk of inadequate monitoring in nonintensive care areas; inadequate physician visits and monitoring of patient; issues of staff knowledge, experience, and training; and problems with alert systems (e.g., not working effectively, staff not responding as required, etc.; Jones, DeVita, and Bellomo 2011). Nurses are involved in all of these areas of care particularly due to their role in surveillance and sharing of information they gain with other health care professionals.

Surveillance in the FTR context is identified in *Keeping Patients Safe* (Child 2004) as a critical aspect of care directly related to nursing care. "Surveillance is monitoring patient status . . . . The goal of surveillance is the early identification and prevention of potential problems, which requires behavioral and cognitive skills" (Child 2004, 91). The effectiveness of surveillance depends on many variables: staff competency, staffing levels, skill mix, communication and interprofessional teams and issues, staff stress levels, staff fatigue, documentation, equipment failure, and more. Additional information about failure modes and effects analysis (FMEA) is available at the IHI website (IHI 2017a).

Rapid Response Teams

The rapid response team (RRT) is a team of health care clinicians (physicians, nurses, respiratory therapists, and others) who are experts in critical care. The team comes to the bedside to assist staff in making rapid decisions when a patient may be experiencing life-threatening complications. The IHI website provides excellent content on RRTs (IHI 2016b). Three system issues that often affect care in critical situations and are connected to the five health care professions core competencies are (IHI 2016b):

1. Failure in planning (including assessment, treatment, patient outcomes);
2. Failure to communicate (patient to staff, staff to patient, staff to physicians, etc.); and

3. Failure to recognize deteriorating patient condition in a timely manner.

Explore how RRTs are used. What impact do RRTs have on staff function? How are these teams used in hospitals? What are the results of using RRTs? How might RRTs affect quality improvement?

Handoffs

Patient transfers are considered high-risk error situations (Child 2004). Transfers can lead to interruptions in care, miscommunications, and duplications of effort. It is common today for patients to move from several care sites, even within the same HCO and during one treatment period such as one hospitalization. For example, patients move from admission through the emergency department to surgery and its various components, to an inpatient unit, and then discharge, which may include rehabilitation, home care, or long-term care.

When do handoffs occur? They occur during transfer from the emergency department to the admitting unit; transfer from one unit to another; when a nurse or physician transfers care to another nurse or physician; transfer to a procedure area; temporary transfer of staff coverage such as for lunch and breaks; transfer from anesthesiologist to the postanesthesia unit; when the primary care provider transfers the patient to hospital staff such as the intensivist, then again during discharge, when the hospital staff transfers the patient back to the primary care provider; transfer to home care or to hospice care; and transfer to a rehab center, long-term care center, or another hospital.

Effective handoffs provide "accurate information about a patient's general care plan, treatment, services, current condition, and any recent or anticipated changes" (Department of Defense [DOD] 2005, 3). Handoffs should support seamless transitions of care, and this requires a systematic, reliable, and efficient system for transmitting information. Handoffs are described as follows (DOD 2005, 3):

- Handoffs are interactive communications providing the opportunity for questioning between the giver and receiver of information about the patient, client, or resident.
- Handoffs include up-to-date information regarding the care, treatment, and services; condition of the patient, client, or resident; and any recent or anticipated changes.
- Interruptions during handoffs are limited to minimize the possibility that information will not be conveyed or will be forgotten.

- Handoffs require a process for verification of the received information, including repeat back or read back, as appropriate.

- The receiver of the handoff information has an opportunity to review relevant patient historical data, which may include previous care, treatment, and services.

Nurses, physicians, and other health care staff are involved in handoffs daily. Nurses have critical roles in handoffs due to the nature of their direct care. You should consider why transfers increase the risk of errors. What are the possible errors that might occur? What is the nurse's role during transfer and how does the nurse consciously prevent errors? What could be changed in the process to reduce risk?

Ambiguity and Workaround Culture

Hospitals are usually organized around functions, and individuals practice in this context. There is, however, often ambiguity regarding responsibility: Who does what when, and how? The health care system naturally experiences breakdowns. How does the staff (individuals and teams) respond to the signs that a breakdown is occurring? Typically, the response is to try to figure out how to get the work done to stay on schedule, without analyzing at that time what is happening and fixing the problem. This response is a *workaround.*

There is a positive aspect of this: many errors are caught before they occur. But the negative result usually is that nothing is learned from the experience and improvement does not occur. There is just relief that an error was avoided and then staff move on. The assumption is that workarounds save time, but many of them do not. "All workers—not just those on the front line—need to be coached to learn how to reduce ambiguity systematically and how to continually improve processes through quick, iterative experiments" (Spear 2005, 85). Using this approach, HCOs learn that they can create more effective, long-term change from small changes. Simulation may be used to experience workarounds and analyzing the experience can help you determine how to best handle workarounds by asking "not what do we need to do to make the process 'better' but rather what specifics prevent us from performing perfectly" (Spear 2005, 88).

Safety in Every Plan of Care

You should include information about safety in patient care plans that you develop. If a standard template is used for care plans it should include safety. Patient safety needs may also change, requiring you to revise the care plan accordingly.

Checklists: A Method to Reduce Wrong-Site Surgery Errors and Other Errors

The ANA has joined more than forty organizations to endorse the use of a new Universal Protocol for Preventing Wrong-Site, Wrong-Procedure and Wrong-Person Surgeries™. More information can be found in the AHRQ patient safety primer on this topic (PSNet 2016b). The protocol includes marking the surgical site, involving the patient in the marking process, and taking a final time-out in the operating room to recheck with the entire team.

Patient Falls

Patient falls are a safety concern for all nurses. The National Database of Nursing Quality Indicators (NDNQI) reports that falls continue to be a problem on all types of units, and approximately 30 percent involve an injury (http://www.pressganey.com/solutions/clinical-quality/nursing-quality; Dunton et al. 2004). The CMS hospital-acquired complications (HACs) initiative also includes falls as a critical problem in health care that is monitored for CMS beneficiaries. Factors to consider in fall risk assessment are history of falls, the environment such as equipment and carpeting, medication use and effects, decreased mental status, decreased mobility, physiological effects of aging, and methods used to call for assistance when the patient is in bed or a chair. Risk variations in patient populations should be noted in appropriate course content, such as care for postsurgery patients, children, older adults, and so on. This assessment should also be addressed in the safety element in care plans.

Infectious Diseases

Infectious diseases are also considered HACs when they are complications, not the reason for admission. You need to know and follow the infection control policies and procedures in the HCOs where you receive clinical experience. Postoperative infections have the most serious consequences of all medical injuries, with increased length of stay, treatment costs, and risk of death. Handwashing is critical and must be reinforced in practice. The Joint Commission also emphasizes handwashing in its accreditation surveys. What should be assessed related to infectious diseases and what are the risks for acquiring and transmitting infectious agents? See the CDC's handwashing guidelines on its website (https://www.cdc.

gov/handwashing/). There are many studies on this problem, providing evidence for best practice (EBP).

Benchmarking

"Benchmarking is an improvement tool whereby a company [or organization] measures its performance or process against other companies' best practices, determines how those companies achieved their performance levels, and uses the information to improve its own performance" (iSix-Sigma 2017a). Many hospitals and other types of HCOs now use benchmarking. One of the popular benchmarking approaches used by HCOs is SixSigma, "a rigorous and a systematic methodology that utilizes information (management by facts) and statistical analysis to measure and improve a company's operational performance, practices, and systems by identifying and preventing 'defects' in manufacturing and service-related processes in order to anticipate and exceed expectations of all stakeholders to accomplish effectiveness" (iSixSigma 2017b).

Assessment of Access to Health Care Services

Access to health care services must be monitored and improved. It is an important element of quality care. *Healthy People 2020* views access to care as a critical need across the country for all types of health care. The Affordable Care Act (ACA) was directed at providing more access to care through greater reimbursement options. When a patient does not have access, the patient's health is at risk and further complications may occur. Access is not a simple concept; for example, it can apply to any of the following:

- Education about when care is needed
- Ability to get an appointment, and in the timeframe needed (for example, appointment times, day of week, wait list)
- Choice of providers
- Access to specialty care when needed
- Transportation to a health care appointment (for example, availability of transportation; funds for transportation)
- Diagnostic tests completed and results reported in a timely manner
- Individual ability to pay for care or availability of an outside source of payment, such as insurance
- Access to a physical facility (e.g., facility with handicap-usable features)
- Access to childcare if needed in order to go to care appointments

- Ability to understand health care information and language (health literacy)

Vulnerable populations (low-income groups; children and adolescents; racial and ethnic minorities; homeless, mentally ill, uninsured, disabled, and elderly people; veterans; immigrants; rural populations; and prisoners) often have limited access. You need to understand the meaning of access to health care, the barriers to access, the impact of lack of access, and the needs of vulnerable populations. You can review the current QDR to learn more about access to care.

Workplace Safety

Workplace safety is a component of health care safety. Why is this important and how does it relate to health care safety? Potential positive effects of workplace safety include:

- Reduced cost of care
- Safer care for patients (a patient may be injured in the same type of incident that injured a nurse)
- Consistent care (reduced risk of sudden nurse absence requiring staff substitution)
- Less stress caused by nursing shortages when staff members are on medical leave due to an injury

See earlier content about staff fatigue, an important topic related to staff safety that also impacts patient safety.

Examples of ANA position statements related to staff safety include *Assuring Patient Safety: The Employer's Role in Promoting Healthy Nursing Work Hours for Registered Nurses in All Roles and Settings, Assuring Patient Safety: Registered Nurses' Responsibility in All Roles and Settings to Guard against Working When Fatigued,* and others. The ANA is a strong advocate for safety for nurses in all types of health care settings. Its position statements on staff safety provide guidelines for work environments. These are excellent resources. Critical staff safety topics include needlesticks, infections, ergonomics (such as Handle with Care®), violence in the workplace, and exposure to chemicals. ANA resources on these and other workplace safety topics are accessible through its website (ANA 2016c).

OSHA and NIOSH

The Occupational Safety and Health Administration (OSHA; https://www. osha.gov/) and the National Institute for Occupational Safety and Health (NIOSH; https://www.cdc.gov/niosh/index.htm) are federal agencies concerned with employee health and safety in all work settings, and both provide resources on staff safety. How do these agencies relate to health care employers and employees? The websites for these agencies provide information about the health risks for specific work settings and strategies used to prevent problems in each. You should understand the worker's compensation system and how it differs from private and other government forms of health insurance. Consider the number of uninsured and underinsured in your state and the impact of unemployment on health care coverage.

CMS Initiative: Hospital-Acquired Conditions

In the fall of 2007, the CMS announced a major change in the inpatient prospective payment system (IPPS) regarding hospital-acquired conditions (HACs). A white paper, *A Summary of the Impact of Reforms to the Hospital Inpatient Prospective Payment System (IPPS) on Nursing Services*, describes the rule change and its effects (Robert Wood Johnson Foundation [RWJF] 2007), and George Washington University School of Nursing adds: "Now, more than ever, hospital leaders need to invest in high-quality nursing care and provide resources to support nurses' ongoing contribution to patient safety and healthcare quality. This rule will have a big effect on how nurses do their jobs" (2007). This change eliminates additional Medicare payments for selected HACs, including inpatient pressure ulcers, certain injuries (for example, fractures from falls), catheter-associated urinary tract infections (CAUTIs), vascular catheter-associated infections, certain surgical-site infections, objects left in during surgery, air embolism, and blood incompatibility. Medicaid is also now a part of this initiative. This change has an impact on HCO finances, which is also important to nursing.

Nursing is involved in the care of patients who experience HACs, and as a consequence, how HCOs respond will involve nursing (RWJF 2007). The worst response would be to decrease the nursing budget to cover the costs of these complications, which will no longer be covered by Medicare or Medicaid. This might lead to reductions in staff and funding for staff education—and neither would be an effective solution. However, this can also be viewed as an opportunity for nursing to demonstrate that it can improve care and control costs: "Reports of nurse-directed interventions that significantly improve the very conditions the payment rule targets have been cited in the literature; risk assessment, surveillance, early diagnosis, treatment, and education have been shown to be effective in lowering rates of pressure ulcers, falls, and infections" (Kurtzman and Buerhaus 2008, 32).

Since the CMS announcement, some insurers have announced that they also will not pay for treating complications on lists they have created. It is not always easy to pinpoint the cause for all of these complications or to determine if they were preventable, so this is likely to lead to some conflicts. This initiative will lead to changes in policies and procedures, increased use of checklists, changes in documentation to improve data, changes in interventions, and increased emphasis on surveillance. Over time, the lists of common HACs will change when data indicate improvement or identify additional problem areas, which means HCOs and health care professionals will need to keep up-to-date.

Transforming Care at the Bedside (TCAB) is one QI initiative that could make a difference in how nursing responds to the CMS ruling on HACs. The TCAB website provides examples of projects that have improved care (IHI 2017c). Chapter 1 includes additional information on TCAB.

You need to understand what is happening with reimbursement for care and complications. This is a good opportunity to link costs, reimbursement, and quality. Medical errors and complications in the United States are expensive. Other issues related to cost and quality are likewise becoming more important. What is the cost of adverse events and inefficient levels of staffing? This question is addressed in a study examining the critical issue of outcomes and costs (Pappas 2008). Nursing costs are a major part of acute care costs, representing at least 50 percent of most hospital budgets. Nurse staffing is a critical element in quality care, and staffing is a major portion of HCO expenses, particularly hospitals. This study "links the occurrence of adverse events to actual patient-level cost per case" (235). Adverse events reflect the level of quality and affect patient outcomes.

Another study examines the effects of the hospital care environment on patient mortality and nurse outcomes: "Staffing and education have well-documented associations with patient outcomes" (Aiken, Clarke, and Sloane 2008, 223). The patient care environment is influenced by factors such as staff education, QI, nurse-manager ability, HCO leadership, support, and collegial nurse-physician relations. The results indicate that when there are better care environments, nurses have more positive job experiences and there are fewer concerns about quality with significantly lower risks of death or failure to rescue.

CMS Initiative: Thirty-Day Unplanned Readmissions

Another new CMS initiative focuses on thirty-day unplanned readmissions, which are defined as any "unplanned readmission to an acute care hospital in the 30 days after discharge" (Medicare.gov 2016). Not only do HCOs need to track and report readmissions, they also need to develop strategies to reduce these readmissions. This should include nurses, as nursing care is directly related to discharge planning and follow-up. Some examples of strategies are medication reconciliation, assessment of discharge needs and development of effective plans with patient and family input, patient education, effective communication, and collaboration with community partners. It is important to note that the responsibility should not just fall on nurses, but on the interprofessional team as a whole. An Institute of Medicine report, *Facilitating Patient Understanding of Discharge Instructions,* provides some guidelines for understanding the impact of health literacy on discharge instructions, and this then relates to problems that may occur that lead to unplanned readmission (Alper and Hernandez 2014). Errors do occur after discharge that may then lead to readmission (PSNet 2016a).

Patients and Families and Quality Improvement

How might patients and families become more involved in the development of safety standards, and why is this important? Explore initiatives to increase patient and family involvement and provide patient resources, such as the National Patient Safety Foundation (NPSF; http://www.npsf.org/?page=patientsandfamilies2), AHRQ patient materials, The Joint Commission Speak Up campaign (https://www.jointcommission.org/speakup.aspx), and the Institute for Safe Medication Practice (http://www.ismp.org/). Staff also need to know how to approach patients and families when errors occur. What might an error mean to a patient or a family? What might they feel (e.g., angry, distrustful of staff, abandoned)? What might be the effect the next time the patient seeks care? Why is it important to ask patients more than just dates of past hospitalizations? A bad past experience can affect current treatment. Put yourself in the place of the patient or family member to gain a better understanding of patient and family responses and how nurses might help them cope. There may be legal ramifications when errors occur.

The Joint Commission and Quality Improvement

What is the purpose of The Joint Commission accreditation and the basic elements of its accreditation process? What are the implications of the professional standards and accreditation? (See discussion in chapter 3.)

The Joint Commission current annual safety goals are now an integral part of HCOs accredited by TJC. You will need to keep informed of changes in the annual goals and in accreditation requirements. HCOs provide ongoing staff education on these topics. Multiple websites provide updates related to standards, guidelines (AHRQ), safety and QI issues, EBP, FDA drug alerts, ANA updates on nursing workforce safety, and the annual QDR.

The Joint Commission standards are available online. These provide you with examples of what is evaluated in the accreditation process. Its website also includes information on patient safety, sentinel events, root cause analysis, performance measurement, and more. The site has a number of current public policy reports on topics such as health literacy and patient safety, organ donation, and community-wide emergency preparedness. These policy statements change as new issues arise.

Access to and Application of Care Management Programs and Guidelines

What care management programs and clinical guidelines are available and where can you access them (e.g., clinical guidelines, patient care protocols, clinical pathways, algorithms, etc.)? These are particularly relevant for patients with chronic problems. Standards, policies, and procedures should be evidence-based, although at this time there is limited research evidence for many nursing care issues. Standards, policies, and procedures for nurses and nursing care should not conflict with regulations (such as the state's nurse practice act) and should conform to nursing standards. HCOs need to ensure that staff members are competent and meet required regulations, especially regarding licensure and credentialing. Faculty need to connect this information to QI and convey this to their students.

How do these programs and guidelines apply to nursing care? The report, *Knowing What Works in Healthcare*, describes the continuum from research studies to systematic review to development of clinical guidelines (Figure S-1, Eden 2008, 23).

Nursing Activities and Relationship to QI

Nurses are very involved in surveillance, which includes assessing or monitoring patients, delivering therapeutic interventions, and coordinating and integrating care from multiple providers (Child 2004). *The Future of Nursing* report (IOM 2011a) describes the need for more nursing leadership in QI, and the earlier report *Keeping Patients Safe* (Child 2004) indicates that nurses are not as prepared as needed to guide QI. You must understand and embrace this QI role. The nurse's role in HCOs is not static; it changes.

The National Quality Strategy (NQS) is now an important part of the national initiative to improve care. Its development was mandated by the ACA (https://www.ahrq.gov/workingforquality/). See earlier discussion on this topic in chapter 2.

What is the ANA NDNQI? What are the issues that the ANA and the American Academy of Nursing (AAN) are investigating through NQF? How oes The Joint Commission use the ANA Report Card? These quality indicators have been linked to patient safety outcomes in such areas as medication errors and falls, and they are also integrated into some electronic medical records and physician order entry systems. In addition, the development and maintenance of the Magnet Recognition Program emphasize QI. Therefore, it seems reasonable that students and faculty should apply these same measures to nursing education. Both of these topics are discussed more in chapter 1.

8

Core Competency: Use Informatics

Communicate, manage knowledge, mitigate error, and support decision-making using informa- tion technology. (Greiner and Knebel 2003, 4)

Use of Computers in Health Care Organizations

Informatics emphasizes the need to manage patient information, protect the patient against errors, and support health care interventions. Health information technology (HIT) is used not only to provide care, but to reduce errors. It is usually an asset in today's health care system, but it can also be problematic: "There is a perception that technology will lead to fewer errors than strategies that focus on staff performance; however, technology may in some circumstances lead to more errors. This is particularly true when technology fails to take into account the end users, increases staff time, replicates an already bad process, or is implemented with insuffi- cient training. The best approach is not always clear, and most approaches have advantages and disadvantages" (Finkelman and Kenner 2007, 55). A 2011 study surveys 16,352 nurses from 316 hospitals in four states about the use of electronic medical records (EMRs) and patient outcomes. The results indicate that the sample believes there has been improvement (Kutney-Lee and Deena 2011). This study is a positive result, and as more health care organizations (HCOs) adopt EMRs, there will likely be more studies assessing the outcomes.

We need to learn how to make HIT safer. According to the Agency for Healthcare Research and Quality (AHRQ), HIT can be effective in providing computerized monitoring of adverse drug events, computer-generated reminders for follow-up testing, computerized provider order entry (CPOE), automated medication dispensers, handheld devices used to access prescription information, EMRs, or electronic health records (EHRs) that can provide portable birth-to-death data, and online support groups for patients (Farley and Battles 2009). In addition, the AHRQ recognizes the need to develop HIT standards in health care and is leading this effort. Computers are generally used in health care for computer-based reminder systems, access to patient information at the point of care, and clinical decision support systems.

At the same time that changes are being made in documentation, incentives are also used to change documentation behavior. In 2008, Medicare began offering physicians incentive payments if they used e-prescriptions (qualified electronic systems that can transmit medication administration) for Medicare patients (Centers for Medicare and Medicaid Services 2014). This program ended in 2013 but e-prescriptions continue to be supported with meaningful use requirements. A barrier to seamless coordination is the lack of interoperable computerized records. To improve information sharing and coordination of care, the percentage of physicians using EMRs and EHRs must increase, and there needs to be greater ability to share between systems. Over time this is expected to occur. The expectation is that the use of EHRs will reach 80 percent by 2016 (Lewis 2011).

Though not all HCOs use the same software, it is critical that you understand the principles of computerized documentation systems. Identifying common errors is also helpful. We need to make technology competencies critical and terminal objectives of our educational programs. *To Err Is Human* emphasizes the need for shared knowledge and the free flow of information, which should be "interactive, real-time, and prospective" (Kohn, Corrigan, and Donaldson 1999, 72). This requires effective use of information technology and students beginning to learn about it in school.

Health Insurance Portability and Accountability Act
The new information infrastructure must meet the requirements of Health Insurance Portability and Accountability Act (HIPAA). How do HIPAA requirements apply to your practice as students as well as after graduation? Use of electronic methods has increased the risk of unauthorized access to health information.

The Digital Divide: Disparities and Informatics

The *digital divide* refers to the problems faced by people with limited access to information technologies (Chang et al. 2004). People with disabilities and low socioeconomic status and rural populations face a barrier between them and the health information and patient-centered care they need. The Health and Medicine Division (HMD) reports make it clear that information technology is critical by making informatics one of the five core health care profession competencies (see chapter 1). *Healthy People 2020* also emphasizes the importance of the Internet in increasing equality. Health literacy is closely tied to informatics as well. Nurses need to understand these issues, recognize the barriers and consider how the barriers might be overcome in communities, and evaluate Internet resources and guide patients in selecting them. Funding is needed to provide more access. Limited access leads to more disparities. Computer literacy is needed across all age groups and for all vulnerable populations. The community should be involved in a plan to improve access.

Computer-Based Reminder Systems and Clinical Decision Support Systems

How do computer-based reminder systems work and how they can assist nurses, such as in reminding nurses of risks for patient falls, allergies, and times for medication or specific required monitoring. If local HCOs include this support in their information technology, consider how it helps staff provide better care.

With today's expanding and rapidly changing knowledge, nurses have a difficult time keeping current. Building this knowledge into information technology to help health care professionals make better decisions should be just as important for nurses as for physicians. You may have installed pharmacology information in your smartphone, tablet, and so on. This is one example of how technology can help in more effective decision-making.

Access to Complete Patient Information at the Point of Care

How can access to patient information at the point of care contribute to nursing? How can you use that information, and how might this eliminate errors and near misses and enhance patient-centered care (PCC)? What devices might be used and by whom to maintain PCC? Using technology in direct care areas should break down barriers to nurse-patient relationships and enhance effective communication.

Meaningful Use

Meaningful use is "the use of certified EHR technology in a meaningful manner (for example electronic prescribing)(CMS 2014); ensuring that the certified EHR technology is connected in a manner that provides for the electronic exchange of health information to improve the quality of care" (CDC 2016c). It is also important to note that when "using certified EHR technology the provider must submit to the Secretary of HHS information on quality of care and other measures" (CDC 2016c). Meaningful use requires that certain criteria are applied to HIT and thus to QI program activities that involve HIT. HIT must (HealthIT.gov 2015):

- "Improve quality, safety, efficiency, and reduce health disparities";
- "Engage patients and family";
- "Improve care coordination, and population and public health"; and
- "Maintain privacy and security of patient health information."

These requirements have changed over time, and in 2016, changes were made based on problems that were identified as needing improvement. Two such changes are putting less focus on rewarding health care providers and HCOs for using HIT and more focus on outcomes, and emphasizing the need to ensure that HIT makes it more straightforward to provide care, not more complicated (Slavitt 2016). The Office of the National Coordinator for Health Information at the CMS is responsible for administration of HIT meaningful use.

Nurses' Involvement in HIT Decisions

Nurses are becoming more involved in HIT development and implementation. The American Academy of Nursing's Workforce Commission, with support from the Robert Wood Johnson Foundation, surveyed nurses and other health care providers at twenty-five sites nationwide about their work processes and environments (Pulley 2008). The results show that there is a need for HIT tools targeting care coordination, care delivery, communications, discharge processes, documentation, medication administration, patient movement, and supplies and equipment management. Nurses indicate that they want all-electronic health records instead of hybrid systems that combine electronic and paper-based reporting; computerized order entry systems to eliminate handwriting legibility issues; touch-screen or voice-activated technology for documentation; and automated networks to collect and download vital patient data. According to the commission's chair, nurses are interested in adding more hands-free tools, particularly wireless technology; greater use of radio-frequency identification technology to track people, supplies, and equipment; robotics to deliver supplies; and smart beds to monitor patient movements, with pressure sensors to reduce the incidence of bedsores. Nurses are important users of HIT and medical technology so nursing must get involved in application design to improve HIT applications (Pulley 2008). Nurses may also be certified in informatics and provide leadership for HIT in a variety of positions.

Many strategies could be used to respond to the need to actively integrate the five health care professions core competencies in nursing education and practice. We need to be creative in our facilitation of learning and encourage greater use of the valuable information and recommendations found in the *Quality Chasm* reports and initiatives that have been developed in response to these reports and their recommendations. We need to also recognize that the HMD continues to work on projects and develop additional expert reports on a variety of health care issues related to the health care professions core competencies, expanding the *Quality Chasm* series. You need to be engaged in learning and preparing for nursing roles and responsibilities and meet the required competencies.

Glossary

Accreditation. The establishment of the status, legitimacy, or appropriateness of an institution, program (for example, composite of modules), or module of study.

Adverse event. Injuries caused by medical management rather than the underlying condition of the patient.

Blame game. A punitive environment that blames an individual for errors.

Care coordination. An interprofessional approach to the care of a patient.

Caregiver. A person who helps in identifying, preventing, or treating illness or disability.

Chronic illness. A long-term or permanent condition.

Clinical judgment. An application of *clinical reasoning*, using in-depth analysis and evaluation of knowledge and skills, whereby the nurse knows why an intervention is needed, is able to perform the intervention competently, and can justify the clinical decision; allowing the clinician to fit his or her knowledge and experience to an individual patient (individual needs, history, and so on).

Clinical reasoning. An in-depth mental process of analysis and evaluation of knowledge and skills; the process of arriving at problem identification (diagnosis).

Coaching. When an expert draws out what the staff or student knows in a bonded clinical situation.

Collaboration. A team approach among health professionals and family to meet patient needs.

Competency. The ability to perform some task and to meet specified qualifications.

Critical thinking. Actively conceptualizing, applying, analyzing, synthesizing, and evaluating information.

Culture of safety. A work culture that focuses on quality from a system perspective rather than focusing on blaming individual staff.

Deep dive. Seeking to improve quality of care by exploring, brainstorming, and prioritizing responses to this critical question: "If you could create the perfect patient and staff experience, what would it look like?"

Delegation. Determining what individual team members should do.

Disclosure of error. Disclosing a harmful medical error, questionable judgment, incident, or misadventure.

Disease management. The coordination and patient-centered use of interventions to decrease length of hospital stay and costs for a disease.

Disparity. Unjustifiable inequality in the treatment of different groups or populations.

Diversity. Racial, cultural, or ethnic variations in the demographics of a place, organization, or profession.

Effective. Designed to provide services with desired outcomes to all who can benefit and refrain from providing services to those not likely to benefit (avoid underuse and overuse, respectively).

Efficient. Designed to avoid waste of equipment, supplies, ideas, energy, or other resources.

Equitable. Designed to provide care that does not vary in quality because of personal characteristics such as gender, ethnicity, geographic location, and socioeconomic status.

Error of omission. An error that occurs because something that should be done is not done.

Error. The failure of a planned action to be completed as intended.

Evidence-based management (EBM). Systematic application of relevant evidence to management decisions to improve performance.

Evidence-based practice (EBP). One of five competencies defined by the Institute of Medicine (IOM); the integration of best clinical practice, research evidence, nursing expertise, and the values and preferences of the individuals, families, and communities served in order to improve patient-centered care.

Failure to rescue (FTR). The avoidable death of a patient.

Family-centered rounds. Nursing rounds that include the patient's family with the patient's consent.

Handoffs. Accurate information about a patient's general care plan, treatment, services, current condition, and any recent or anticipated changes provided by one health care provider to another when the patient changes physical location (such as from one unit to another) or changes health care providers.

Health care disparity. Unjustifiable inequality in the health care of different groups or populations.

Health informatics technology (HIT). One of five competencies defined by the IOM; to communicate, manage knowledge, mitigate error, and support decision-making using information technology.

Health literacy. The degree to which individuals have the capacity to obtain, process, and understand basic information and services needed to make appropriate decisions regarding their health.

High-fidelity simulation equipment. Use of mannequins (human simulators) or equipment common to a particular clinical situation to allow the learner to repeatedly practice appropriate skills in an environment as close to reality as possible.

Indicator. A measurement used to assess health care structure, process, or outcomes.

Integrative review. Systematic summaries of appraised studies to provide EBP evidence; a form of EBP literature.

Interdisciplinary or interprofessional teams. One of five competencies defined by the IOM; health care professionals from several fields cooperating, collaborating, communicating, and integrating care in teams to ensure that care is continuous and reliable.

Interprofessional education (IPE). Joint teaching and learning of students from different professions in order to promote collaborative working in their professional practice.

Just culture. A nonpunitive, fair, and just system that includes personal and professional accountability for one's practice and for actively improving the processes of care, focusing more on system issues and errors rather than individual staff.

Latent failures. Systems faults that allow or fail to stop errors.

Medication administration record (MAR). Computer-generated schedule for administering medications to a patient for a defined period, including physician's orders and time of day to administer the agents.

Medication reconciliation. Creating the most accurate list possible of all medications a patient is taking—including drug name, dosage, frequency, and route—and comparing that list against the physician's admission, transfer, and discharge orders with the goal of providing correct medications to the patient at all transition points within the hospital.

Misuse. Improperly applying treatments to a patient.

Near miss. An error that was caught before it could occur.

Nurse externship. A program designed to increase the clinical confidence and competence of nursing students, in which they work under the direct supervision of a registered nurse supervisor; usually occurs between the junior and senior years.

Nurse residency. A program designed to transition the nurse from a student to professional nurse.

Outcome. The effects on health status that are attributable to a planned intervention or series of interventions.

Overuse. Providing more care than needed.

Palliative care. Appropriate and compassionate care provided for patients with life-limiting illnesses.

Patient-centered care. One of five competencies defined by the IOM for health care professionals; an approach to the planning, delivery, and evaluation of health care to provide better outcomes that includes the patient and their individual preferences.

Patient-centered rounds. Regular patient visits in which health care professionals are careful to provide medical information to the patient, answer questions, and involve the patient in decisions.

Plan, Do, Study, Act (PDSA). A continuous quality improvement model consisting of a logical sequence of four repeated steps: Plan, Do, Study (or Check), and Act.

Process. Methods or functions that are used to achieve an outcome.

Quality improvement (QI). One of five competencies defined by the IOM for health care professionals; identifying errors and hazards in care, understanding and implementing basic safety design principles such as standardization and simplification, understanding and continually measuring care quality in terms of structure, process, and outcomes in relation to patient and community needs, and designing and testing interventions to change processes and systems of care, with the objective of improving quality; often also referred to as continuous quality improvement (CQI) to emphasize that it is ongoing.

Quality. The degree to which health services for individuals and populations increase the likelihood of desired health outcomes and are consistent with current professional knowledge; consists of structure, process, and outcome elements.

Rapid response team (RRT). A team of health care clinicians (physicians, nurses, respiratory therapists, etc.) and experts in critical care who come to the bedside to assist staff in making rapid decisions when a patient is in trouble.

Research. Systematic study directed toward fuller scientific knowledge or understanding of the subject.

Root cause analysis. A method designed to examine the causes of an adverse patient event.

Safety. The avoidance of injury or harm when providing care.

Safety net hospitals. Hospitals that serve a large number of vulnerable patients who have inadequate or no health care coverage and poor access to health care services.

Self-management. Acceptance by the patient of much of the responsibility for the patient's own care, such as adhering to a prescribed medical regimen or regulating his or her lifestyle.

Sentinel event. An unanticipated event in a health care setting that results in death or serious physical or psychological injury to a person, not related to the natural course of the patient's illness.

Simulation. Replication of clinical experiences in a safe environment as part of a student's education.

Surveillance. Monitoring patient status with the goals of early identification and prevention of problems.

Systematic review. A summary of all the published research relevant to a specific question or topic.

Timely. Involving a minimum of waiting or delay for both patients and caregivers.

Underuse. An adverse event caused by failure to provide appropriate care rather than the underlying condition of the patient.

Workaround. A rushed, improvised response to a breakdown in a work process, made without pausing to analyze and correct the underlying problem.

Acronyms & Abbreviations

AACN: American Association of Colleges of Nursing

ADE: adverse drug event

ADN: Associate Degree Nurse; Associate Degree Nursing (program)

AHRQ: Agency for Healthcare Research and Quality

ANA: American Nurses Association

ANCC: American Nurses Credentialing Center

AONE: American Organization of Nurse Executives

APRN: advanced practice registered nurse

BSN: Bachelor of Science in Nursing [degree]

CDC: Centers for Disease Control and Prevention

CER: comparative effectiveness research

CMS: Centers for Medicare and Medicaid Services

CNL: Clinical Nurse-Leader

CPG: clinical practice guideline

CPOE: computerized physician order entry

CPOES: computerized point-of-entry system

CQI: continuing quality improvement

DEU: dedicated education unit

DNP: Doctor of Nursing Practice [degree]

EBM: evidence-based management

EBP: evidence-based practice

EHR: electronic health record

EMR: electronic medical record

EMTALA: Emergency Medical Treatment and Labor Act

FDA: Food and Drug Administration

FMEA: failure modes and effects analysis

FTR: failure to rescue

HAC: hospital-acquired complication/condition

HCO: health care organization

HDM: Health and Medicine Division [since 2015; formerly Institute of Medicine]

HHS: Department of Health and Human Services

HIPAA: Health Insurance Portability and Accountability Act

HIT: health informatics technology

HRSA: Health Resources and Services Administration

IHI: Institute for Healthcare Improvement

IOM: Institute of Medicine [through early 2015; now Health and Medicine Division]

IPE: interprofessional education

IPEC: Interprofessional Education Collaborative

ISMP: Institute for Safe Medication Practices

MAR: medication administration record

MSN: Master of Science in Nursing [degree]

NASEM: National Academies of Sciences, Engineering, and Medicine; also known as "the National Academies"

NCCMERP: National Coordinating Council for Medication Error Reporting and Prevention

NCNQ: National Center for Nursing Quality®

NCSBN: National Council of State Boards of Nursing

NDNQI: National Database of Nursing Quality Indicators®

NIH: National Institutes of Health

NINR: National Institute of Nursing Research

NIOSH: National Institute for Occupational Safety and Health

NLN: National League for Nursing

NQF: National Quality Forum

NQS: National Quality Strategy

OSHA: Occupational and Safety Health Administration

PCC: patient-centered care

PCORI: Patient-Centered Outcomes Research Institute

PDSA: Plan, Do, Study, Act

PHR: personal health record

QDR: National Healthcare Quality and Disparities Report

QI: quality improvement

QSEN: Quality and Safety Education for Nurses

RCT: randomized clinical/controlled trial

RN: registered nurse

RRT: rapid response team

RWJF: Robert Wood Johnson Foundation

SBAR: Situation-Background-Assessment-Recommendation

SIRC: Simulation Innovation Resource Center

TCAB: Transforming Care at the Bedside

TERCAP: Taxonomy of Error, Root Cause Analysis, and Practice Responsibility

UAP: unlicensed assistive personnel

WHO: World Health Organization

References

Abelson, R., and M. Sanger-Katz. 2016. "Obamacare Obstacles and Some Possible Solutions." *New York Times*, August 30, pp. B1, B8.

Ackroyd-Stolarz, S., N. Hartnell, and N. MacKinnon. 2005. "Approaches to Improving the Safety of the Medication Use System." *Healthcare Quarterly* 8 (Spec. no.): 59–64.

Adams, K., and J. Corrigan, eds. 2003. *Priority Areas for National Action: Transforming Health Care Quality*. Washington, DC: National Academies Press.

Adler, N., and A. Page, eds. 2007. *Cancer Care for the Whole Patient: Meeting Psychosocial Health Needs*. Washington, DC: National Academies Press.

Advisory Commission on Consumer Protection and Quality in the Healthcare Industry. 1999. *Quality First: Better Health Care for All Americans*. Washington, DC: US Government Printing Office.

Agency for Healthcare Research and Quality. 2015. *2014 National Healthcare Quality and Disparities Report*. Rockville, MD: Agency for Healthcare Research and Quality.

———. 2016. "Health Literacy Measurement Tools (Revised)." Quality & Patient Safety. http://www.ahrq.gov/professionals/quality-patient-safety/quality-resources/tools/literacy/index.html.

———. 2017a. "About the National Quality Strategy." https://www.ahrq.gov/workingforquality/about.htm.

———. 2017b. National Quality Strategy Stakeholder Toolkit. Retrieved from https://www.ahrq.gov/sites/default/files/wysiwyg/nqstoolkit2016.pdf.

Aiken, L., S. Clarke, and D. Sloane. 2008. "Effects of Hospital Care Environment on Patient Mortality and Nurse Outcomes." *Journal of Nursing Administration* 38 (5): 223–29.

Alexander, M., C. Durham, J. Hooper, P. Jeffries, N. Goldman, S. Kardong-Edgren, K. Kesten et al. 2015. "NCSBN Simulation Guidelines for Prelicensure Programs." *Journal of Nursing Regulation* 6 (3): 39–42.

Alper, J., ed. 2015a. *Health Literacy: Past, Present, and Future: Workshop and Summary*. Washington, DC: National Academies Press.

———, ed. 2015b. *Informed Consent and Health Literacy: Workshop Summary*. Washington, DC: National Academies Press.

———, ed. 2016a. *Health Literacy and Palliative Care: Workshop Summary*. Washington, DC: National Academies Press.

———, ed. 2016b. *Relevance of Health Literacy to Precision Medicine: Proceedings of a Workshop*. Washington, DC: National Academies Press.

Alper, J., and L. Hernandez, eds. 2014. *Facilitating Patient Understanding of Discharge Instructions: Workshop Summary.* Washington, DC: National Academies Press. https://www.nap.edu/read/18834/chapter/1.

Altman, S., A. Stith Butler, and L. Shern, eds. 2016. *Assessing Progress on the Institute of Medicine Report "The Future of Nursing".* Washington, DC: National Academies Press.

American Association of Colleges of Nursing. 2006. *The Essentials of Doctoral Education for Advanced Nursing Practice.* Washington, DC: American Association of Colleges of Nursing.

———. 2008a. *Cultural Competency in Baccalaureate Nursing Education.* Washington, DC: American Association of Colleges of Nursing. http://www.aacn.nche.edu/Education/pdf/competency.pdf.

———. 2008b. *The Essentials of Baccalaureate Education for Professional Nursing Practice.* Washington, DC: American Association of Colleges of Nursing.

———. 2008c. *Tool Kit of Resources for Cultural Competent Education for Baccalaureate Nurses.* http://www.aacn.nche.edu/education-resources/toolkit.pdf.

———. 2011a. *The Essentials of Masters Education in Nursing.* Washington, DC: American Association of Colleges of Nursing.

———. 2011b. *Tool Kit for Cultural Competence in Master's and Doctoral Nursing Education.* http://www.aacn.nche.edu/education-resources/Cultural_Competency_Toolkit_Grad.pdf.

———. 2012. "Expectations for Practice Experiences in the RN to Baccalaureate Curriculum." White Paper. http://www.aacn.nche.edu/aacn-publications/white-papers/RN-BSN-White-Paper.pdf.

———. 2015a. "Accelerated Entry-Level Baccalaureate and Master's Degrees in Nursing." Fact Sheet. http://www.aacn.nche.edu/media-relations/fact-sheets/accelerated-programs.

———. 2015b. "Creating a More Qualified Nursing Workforce." Fact Sheet. http://www.aacn.nche.edu/media-relations/fact-sheets/nursing-workforce.

———. 2015c. *The Doctor of Nursing Practice: Current Issues and Clarifying Recommendations.* Report from the Task Force on the Implementation of the DNP, August. http://www.aacn.nche.edu/aacn-publications/white-papers/DNP-Implementation-TF-Report-8-15.pdf.

———. 2015d. "Nursing Faculty Shortage Fact Sheet." http://www.aacn.nche.edu/media-relations/FacultyShortageFS.pdf.

———. 2016a. *Advancing Healthcare Transformation: A New Era for Academic Nursing.* Washington, DC: American Association of Colleges of Nursing. http://www.aacn.nche.edu/AACN-Manatt-Report.pdf.

———. 2016b. "The Changing Landscape: Nursing Student Diversity on the Rise." Policy Brief. http://www.aacn.nche.edu/government-affairs/Student-Diversity-FS.pdf.

American Association of Colleges of Nursing and Association of American Medical Colleges. 2010. *Lifelong Learning in Medicine and Nursing.* Washington, DC: American Association of Colleges of Nursing. www.aacn.nche.edu/education-resources/MacyReport.pdf.

American College of Emergency Physicians. 2011. "The Uninsured: Access to Medical Care." https://www.acep.org/content.aspx?id=45983.

American College of Physicians Foundation. 2007. "Improving Prescription Drug Container Labeling in the United States: A Health Literacy and Medication Safety Initiative." White paper presented at the Institute of Medicine Roundtable on Health Literacy, October 12. http://nationalacademies.org/hmd/~/media/Files/Activity%20Files/PublicHealth/HealthLiteracy/Commissioned-Papers/Improving%20Prescription%20Drug%20Container%20Labeling%20in%20the%20United%20States.pdf.

American Nurses Association. 2015a. *Code of Ethics for Nurses with Interpretive Statements.* Silver Spring, MD: American Nurses Association.

———. 2015b. *Nursing Informatics: Scope and Standards of Practice.* 2nd ed. Silver Spring, MD: American Nurses Association.

———. 2015c. *Nursing: Scope and Standards of Practice.* 3rd ed. Silver Spring, MD: American Nurses Association.

———. 2016a. "2016 Culture of Safety." http://nursingworld.org/MainMenuCategories/ThePracticeofProfessionalNursing/2016-Culture-of-Safety.

———. 2016b. "Healthy Nurse, Healthy Nation™." http://nursingworld.org/MainMenuCategories/WorkplaceSafety/Healthy-Nurse.

———. 2016c. "Healthy Work Environment." http://nursingworld.org/MainMenuCategories/WorkplaceSafety/Healthy-Work-Environment.

———. 2016d. "Nurse Fatigue." http://www.nursingworld.org/MainMenuCategories/WorkplaceSafety/Healthy-Work-Environment/Work-Environment/NurseFatigue.

———. 2016e. *Nursing Administration: Scope and Standards of Practice.* 2nd ed. Silver Spring, MD: American Nurses Association.

———. 2016f. "Work Environment." http://nursingworld.org/MainMenuCategories/WorkplaceSafety/Healthy-Work-Environment/Work-Environment.

American Nurses Credentialing Center. 2013a. *Empirical Outcomes: Criteria for Nursing Excellence.* Silver Spring, MD: American Nurses Credentialing Center.

———. 2013b. *Exemplary Professional Practice: Criteria for Nursing Excellence.* Silver Spring, MD: American Nurses Credentialing Center.

———. 2013c. *New Knowledge, Innovations, & Improvements: Criteria for Nursing Excellence.* Silver Spring, MD: American Nurses Credentialing Center.

———. 2013d. *Structural Empowerment: Criteria for Nursing Excellence.* Silver Spring, MD: American Nurses Credentialing Center.

————. 2013e. *Transformational Leadership: Criteria for Nursing Excellence*. Silver Spring, MD: American Nurses Credentialing Center.

American Organization of Nurse Executives. 2012. "AONE Strategic Plan." www.aone. org/membership/about/docs/2012-2014.AONE.StratPlan.FINAL.doc.

Anderson, K., and S. Olson, eds. 2015. *Achieving Health Equity via the Affordable Care Act: Provisions, and Making Reform a Reality for Diverse Patients: Workshop Summary*. Washington, DC: National Academies Press.

————, eds. 2016. *The Promises and Perils of Digital Strategies in Achieving Health Equity: Workshop Summary*. Washington, DC: National Academies Press.

Aspden, P., ed. 2006. *Preventing Medication Errors*. Washington, DC: National Academies Press.

Aspden, P., J. Corrigan, J. Wolcott, and S. Erickson, eds. 2004. *Patient Safety: Achieving a New Standard of Care*. Washington, DC: National Academies Press.

Association of American Medical Colleges. 2008. *The Medical Home*. AAMC Position Statement. https://members.aamc.org/eweb/upload/The%20Medical%20Home. pdf.

Balogh, E., B. Miller, and J. Ball, eds. 2015. *Improving Diagnosis in Health Care*. Washington, DC: National Academies Press.

Banister, G., L. Butt, and R. Hackel. 1996. "How Nurses Perceive Medication Errors." *Nursing Management* 27 (1): 31–34.

Banja, J. 2005. *Medical Errors and Medical Narcissism*. Sudbury, MA: Jones & Bartlett Learning.

Barnsteiner, J., J. Disch, L. Hall, D. Mayer, and S. Moore. 2007. "Promoting Inter-Professional Education." *Nursing Outlook* 55 (3): 144–50.

Batalden, P. 1998. *Eight Knowledge Domains for Health Professional Students*. Institute for Healthcare Improvement. http://www.ihi.org/education/ihiopenschool/ resources/Assets/Publications%20-%20EightKnowledgeDomainsforHealth ProfessionalStudents_5216cd8e-1867-4c77-90b6-955641ecab78/Knowledge Domains.pdf

Behrman, R., and A. Stith Butler, eds. 2007. *Preterm Birth: Causes, Consequences, and Prevention*. Washington, DC: National Academies Press.

Benner, P. 2001. *From Novice to Expert*. Commemorative ed. Upper Saddle River, NJ: Prentice Hall Health.

Benner, P., M. Sutphen, V. Leonard, and L. Day. 2010. *Educating Nurses: A Call for Radical Transformation*. San Francisco: Jossey-Bass.

Berwick, D. 2008. "The Science of Improvement." *Journal of the American Medical Association* 299 (10): 1182–84.

Berwick, D., A. Downey, and E. Cornett, eds. 2016. *A National Trauma Care System: Integrating Military and Civilian Trauma Systems to Achieve Zero Preventable Deaths after Injury*. Washington, DC: National Academies Press.

Betancourt, J., A. Green, J. Carrillo, and E. Park. 2005. "Cultural Competence and Health Care Disparities: Key Perspectives and Trends." *Health Affairs* 24:499–505.

Blumenthal, D., E. Malphrus, and J. M. McGinnis, eds. 2015. *Vital Signs: Core Metrics for Health and Health Care Progress.* Washington, DC: National Academies Press.

Boysen, Philip G. 2013. "Just Culture: A Foundation for Balanced Accountability and Patient Safety." *Ochsner Journal* 13 (3): 400–406.

Burstin, H., S. Leatherman, and D. Goldmann. 2016. "The Evolution of Healthcare Quality Measurement in the United States." *Journal of Internal Medicine* 279 (2): 154–59.

Campinha-Bacote, J., D. Claymore-Cuny, D. Cora-Bramble, J. Gilbert, R. M. Husbands, R. C. Like, R. Llerena-Quinn et al. 2005. *Transforming the Face of Health Professions through Cultural and Linguistic Competence Education: The Role of the HRSA Centers of Excellence.* Rockville, MD: US Department of Health and Human Services. https://www.researchgate.net/profile/Robert_Like/publication/228998699_Transforming_the_face_of_health_professions_through_cultural_and_linguistic_competence_education_The_role_of_the_HRSA_Centers_of_Excellence/links/00463522667ce19e4e000000.pdf.

Centers for Disease Control and Prevention. 2014. "The Public Health System and the Ten Essential Public Health Services." National Public Health Performance Standards. http://www.cdc.gov/nphpsp/essentialServices.html.

———. 2016a. "Bullying Research." http://www.cdc.gov/violenceprevention/youthviolence/bullyingresearch/index.html.

———. 2016b. "Chronic Disease Overview." http://www.cdc.gov/chronicdisease/overview/.

———. 2016c. "Meaningful Use." http://www.cdc.gov/ehrmeaningfuluse/introduction.html.

Centers for Medicare and Medicaid Services. 2007. CMS rule limiting payment for avoidable complications has big implications for nurses. https://www.medicaid.gov/Federal-Policy-Guidance/downloads/SMD073108.pdf.

———. 2014. "Electronic Prescribing (eRx) Incentive Program." January 1. https://www.cms.gov/Medicare/Quality-Initiatives-Patient-Assessment-Instruments/ERxIncentive/.

———. 2015. *CMS Quality Improvement Roadmap.* https://www.cms.gov/Medicare/Coverage/CouncilonTechInnov/downloads/qualityroadmap.pdf.

———. 2016. "Hospital-Acquired Condition Reduction Program (HACRP)." December 22. https://www.cms.gov/Medicare/Medicare-Fee-for-Service-Payment/AcuteInpatientPPS/HAC-Reduction-Program.html.

Chang, B., S. Bakken, S. S. Brown, T. Houston, G. Kreps, R. Kukafka, C. Safran, and Z. Stavri. 2004. "Bridging the Digital Divide: Reaching Vulnerable Populations." *Journal of the American Medical Informatics Association* 11 (6): 448–57. doi:10.1197/jamia.M1535.

Chao, S., ed. 2007a. *Advancing Quality Improvement Research: Challenges and Opportunities – Workshop Summary.* Washington, DC: National Academies Press.

———, ed. 2007b. *The State of QI and Implementation Research.* Washington, DC: National Academies Press.

Chassin, M., and R. Galvin. 1998. "The Urgent Need to Improve Healthcare Quality." *Journal of the American Medical Association* 280 (2): 1000–1005.

Child, A., ed. 2004. *Keeping Patients Safe: Transforming the Work Environment of Nurses.* Washington, DC: National Academies Press.

Clarke, S., and L. Aiken. 2003. "Failure to Rescue." *American Journal of Nursing* 103 (1): 42–47.

Corrigan, J., J. Eden, and B. Smith, eds. 2003. *Leadership By Example: Coordinating Government Roles in Improving Healthcare Quality.* Washington, DC: National Academies Press.

Craig, C., D. Eby, and J. Whittington. 2011. *Care Coordination Model: Better Care at Lower Cost for People with Multiple Health and Social Needs.* IHI Innovation Series white paper. Boston: Institute for Healthcare Improvement.

Cuff, P., ed. 2014a. *Assessing Health Professional Education: Workshop Summary.* Washington, DC: National Academies Press.

———, ed. 2014b. *Building Health Workforce Capacity through Community-Based Health Professional Education: Workshop Summary.* Washington, DC: National Academies Press.

———, ed. 2016. *Envisioning the Future of Health Professional Education: Workshop Summary.* Washington, DC: National Academies Press.

Daschle, T., J. Lambrew, and S. Greenberger. 2008. *Critical: What We Can Do about the Health-Care Crisis.* New York: Thomas Dunne Books.

Davies, D., M. Davis, A. Jadad, L. Perrier, D. Rath, D. Ryan, G. Sibbald et al. 2003. "The Case for Knowledge Translation: Shortening the Journey from Evidence to Effect." *British Medical Journal* 327 (7405): 33–35.

Dekker, S. 2007. *Just Culture: Balancing Safety and Accountability.* Burlington, VT: Ashgate.

Department of Defense. 2005. "Patient Safety Program." In *Healthcare Communications Toolkit to Improve Transitions in Care.* Washington, DC: Department of Defense.

Department of Health and Human Services. 2012. "Educational and Community-Based Programs." Healthy People 2020. http://healthypeople.gov/2020/topics objectives2020/overview.aspx?topicid=11.

———. 2015. "HHS Strategic Plan: Strategic Plan FY 2014 - 2018." http://www.hhs. gov/about/strategic-plan/index.html.

DeWalt, C., N. Berkman, S. Sheridan, K. Lohr, and M. Pignone. 2004. "Literacy and Health Outcomes: A Systematic Review of the Literature." *Journal of General Internal Medicine* 19 (12): 1228–39.

DeWalt, D., and M. Pignone. 2008. "Advocacy and Patient Literacy: What Healthcare Professionals Can Do to Help Patients Overcome Patient Literacy Barriers." In Earp, French, and Gilkey, *Patient Advocacy*, 215–39.

Dickson, G., and L. Flynn. 2012. "Nurses' Clinical Reasoning: Processes and Practices of Medication Safety." *Qualitative Health Research* 22 (1): 3–16.

Donabedian, A. 1980. *Explorations in Quality Assessment and Monitoring.* Vol. 1, *The Definition of Quality and Approaches to Its Assessment*. Ann Arbor, MI: Health Administration Press.

———. 1996. "Evaluating the Quality of Medical Care." *Milbank Quarterly* 44:166–203.

Draper, D., L. Felland, A. Liebhaber, and L. Melichar. 2008. "The Role of Nurses in Hospital Quality Improvement." *HSC Research Brief*, no. 3, March. http://www.hschange.org/CONTENT/972/.

Dunton, N., B. Gajewski, R. Taunton, and J. Moore. 2004. "Nursing Staffing and Patient Falls in Acute Care Hospital Units." *Nursing Outlook* 52 (1): 53–59.

Earp, J., E. French, and M. Gilkey, eds. 2008. *Patient Advocacy for Healthcare Quality.* Boston: Jones & Bartlett Learning.

Eden, J., ed. 2008. *Knowing What Works in Health Care: A Roadmap for the Nation.* Washington, DC: National Academies Press.

Eden, J., L. Levit, A. Berg, and S. Morton, eds. 2011. *Finding What Works in Health Care: Standards for Systematic Reviews*. Washington, DC: National Academies Press.

Ein Lewin, M., and S. Altman, eds. 2000. *America's Health Care Safety Net: Intact but Endangered*. Washington, DC: National Academies Press.

England, M., A. Stith Butler, and M. Gonzalez, eds. 2015. *Psychosocial Interventions for Mental and Substance Use Disorders: A Framework for Establishing Evidence-Based Standards*. Washington, DC: National Academies Press.

Enthoven, A. 2008. "Healthcare with a Few Bucks Left Over." *New York Times*, December 28, p. WK9.

Farley, D. O., and J. B. Battles. 2009. "Evaluation of the AHRQ Patient Safety Initiative: Framework and Approach." *Health Services Research* 44 (2): 628–45.

Ferguson, B. 2008. "Health Literacy and Health Disparities: The Role They Play in Maternal Child Health." *Nursing for Women's Health* 12 (4): 286–98.

Fineberg, H. 2012. "A Successful and Sustainable Health System—How to Get There from Here." *New England Journal of Medicine* 366 (11): 1020–27.

Finkelman, A. 2011. *Case Management for Nurses*. Saddle Brook, NJ: Pearson Education.

Finkelman, A., and C. Kenner. 2007. "Commentary: Why Should Nurse Leaders Care about the Status of Nursing Education?" *Nurse Leader* 5 (6): 23–27.

Foley, M., and H. Gelband, eds. 2001. *Improving Palliative Care for Cancer: Summary and Recommendations*. Washington, DC: National Academies Press.

Fowler, M. 2015a. *Guide to the Code of Ethics for Nurses with Interpretive Statements.* 2nd ed. Silver Spring, MD: American Nurses Association.

———. 2015b. *Guide to Nursing's Social Policy Statement: Understanding the Profession from Social Contract to Social Covenant.* Silver Spring, MD: American Nurses Association.

Gallagher, R., and D. Nadzam, eds. 2015. *Two Decades of Coordinating Medication Safety Efforts.* National Coordinating Council for Medication Error Reporting and Prevention. http://www.nccmerp.org/sites/default/files/20_year_report.pdf.

Gaskill, M. 2008. "Learning from Mistakes: 'Just Culture' Is Replacing Blame in Some California Hospitals." *NurseWeek (California)* 21 (8): 14–15.

Gebbie, K., L. Rosenstock, and L. Hernandez, eds. 2003. *Who Will Keep the Public Healthy? Educating Public Health Professionals for the 21st Century.* Washington, DC: The National Academies Press.

George Washington University School of Nursing. 2007. "CMS Rule Limiting Payment for Avoidable Complications Has Big Implications for Nurses." November 13. https://nursing.gwu.edu/cms-rule-limiting-payment-avoidable-complications-has-big-implications-nurses.

Gindi, R., L. Black, and R. Cohen. 2016. "Reasons for Emergency Room Use among U.S. Adults Aged 18–64: National Health Interview Survey 2013 and 2014." *National Health Statistics Reports* no. 90, February 18. http://www.cdc.gov/nchs/data/nhsr/nhsr090.pdf.

Glassman, K., and P. Rosenfeld. 2015. *Data Makes a Difference: The Smart Nurse's Handbook for Using Data to Improve Care.* Silver Spring, MD: American Nurses Association.

Gleason, K., H. Brake, V. Agramonte, and C. Perfetti. 2011. *Medications at Transitions and Clinical Handoffs (MATCH) Toolkit for Medication Reconciliation.* AHRQ Publication No. 11(12)-0059. Rockville, MD: Agency for Healthcare Research and Quality. https://www.ahrq.gov/sites/default/files/publications/files/match.pdf.

Gold, D., S. Rogacz, N. Bock, T. Tosteson, T. Baum, F. Speizer, and C. Czeisler. 1992. "Rotating Shift-Work, Sleep and Accidents Related to Sleepiness in Hospital Nurses." *American Journal of Public Health* 82 (7): 1011–14.

Gordon, S. 2005. *Nursing Against the Odds.* Ithaca: Cornell University Press.

Grady, P. A. 2016. "Director's Message: NINR's Strategic Plan: Advancing Science, Improving Lives." NINR. https://www.ninr.nih.gov/aboutninr/directors-message/directors-message.

Graham, R., ed. 2011. *Clinical Practice Guidelines We Can Trust.* Washington, DC: National Academies Press.

Graham, R., M. McCoy, and A. Schultz, eds. 2015. *Strategies to Improve Cardiac Arrest Survival: A Time to Act.* Washington, DC: National Academies Press.

Greiner, A., and E. Knebel, eds. 2003. *Health Professions Education: A Bridge to Quality*. Washington, DC: National Academies Press.

Guidry, M., T. Vischi, R. Han, and O. Passons. 2010. *Healthy People in Healthy Communities*. N.p.: Office of Disease Prevention and Health Promotion. http://www.healthypeople.gov/2010/publications/healthycommunities2001/healthycom01hk.pdf.

Harding, L., and T. Petrick. 2008. "Nursing Student Medication Errors: A Retrospective Review." *Journal of Nursing Education* 47 (1): 43–47.

Harper, M. G., and P. Maloney, eds. 2016. *Nursing Professional Development: Scope and Standards of Practice*. 3rd ed. Chicago: Association for Nursing Professional Development.

Harris, R. 2016. "Reviews of Medical Studies May Be Tainted By Funders' Influence." *Shots: Health News from NPR*, October 12. http://www.npr.org/sections/health-shots/2016/10/12/497550681/reviews-of-medical-studies-may-be-tainted-by-funders-influence.

Health and Medicine Division. 2015a. *Healthy, Resilient, and Sustainable Communities after Disasters: Strategies, Opportunities, and Planning for Recovery*. Washington, DC: National Academies Press.

———. 2015b. *Sharing Clinical Trial Data: Maximizing Benefits, Minimizing Risk*. Washington, DC: National Academies Press.

———. 2016a. "About HMD." National Academies. http://www.nationalacademies.org/hmd/About-HMD.aspx.

———. 2016b. *Collaboration between Health Care and Public Health: Workshop Summary*. Washington, DC: National Academies Press.

———. 2016c. *A Framework for Educating Health Professionals to Address the Social Determinants of Health. Washington, DC: National Academies Press.*

HealthIT.gov. 2010. "Meaningful Use Definition & Objectives." https://www.healthit.gov/providers-professionals/meaningful-use-definition-objectives.

Health Resources and Services Administration. 2010. "HRSA Study Finds Nursing Workforce Is Growing and More Diverse." Press release, March 17. https://www.hrsa.gov/about/news/pressreleases/2010/100317_hrsa_study_100317_finds_nursing_workforce_is_growing_and_more_diverse.html.

Healthcare Information and Management Systems Society. 2015. *2015 Impact of the Informatics Nurse Survey*. http://www.himss.org/ni-impact-survey.

Hernandez, L., ed. 2009. *Health Literacy, eHealth, and Communication: Putting the Consumer First: Workshop Summary*. Washington, DC: National Academies Press.

Hernandez, L., and S. Landi, eds. 2011. *Promoting Health Literacy to Encourage Prevention and Wellness: Workshop Summary*. Washington, DC: National Academies Press.

Hewitt, M., and P. A. Ganz, eds. 2006. *From Cancer Patient to Cancer Survivor: Lost in Transition.* Washington, DC: National Academies Press.

Hewitt, M., and L. Hernandez, eds. 2014. *Implications of Health Literacy in Public Health: Workshop Summary.* Washington, DC: National Academies Press.

Hughes, R., and E. Ortiz. 2005. "Medication Errors: Why They Happen, and How They Can Be Prevented." *American Journal of Nursing* 105 (suppl. 3): 14–23.

Hughes, R., and A. Rogers. 2004. "Are You Tired? Sleep Deprivation Compromises Nurses' Health—and Jeopardizes Patients." *American Journal of Nursing* 104 (3): 15.

Hurtado, M., E. Swift, and J. Corrigan, eds. 2001. *Envisioning the National Healthcare Quality Report.* Washington, DC: National Academies Press.

Improving Chronic Illness Care. 2003. "The Chronic Care Model." http://www.improvingchroniccare.org/index.php?p=The_Chronic_Care_Model&s=2.

Institute for Healthcare Improvement. 2008a. "A New Era in Nursing: Transforming Care at the Bedside." Brochure. http://www.rwjf.org/en/library/research/2007/04/a-new-era-in-nursing.html.

———. 2008b. "Self-Management Support." http://www.ihi.org/IHI/Topics/PatientCenteredCare/SelfManagementSupport/.

———. 2011. "Transforming Care at the Bedside." Program Results Report, July 11. http://www.rwjf.org/en/library/research/2011/07/transforming-care-at-the-bedside.html.

———. 2014. "Partnering in Self-Management Support: A Toolkit for Clinicians." Cambridge, MA: Institute for Healthcare Improvement. http://www.ihi.org/resources/Pages/Tools/SelfManagementToolkitforClinicians.aspx.

———. 2016a. "Changes to Improve Chronic Care." http://www.ihi.org/resources/Pages/Changes/ChangestoImproveChronicCare.aspx.

———. 2016b. "Rapid Response Teams." http://www.ihi.org/Topics/RapidResponseTeams/Pages/default.aspx.

———. 2017a. "Failure Modes and Effects Analysis (FMEA) Tool." http://www.ihi.org/resources/Pages/Tools/FailureModesandEffectsAnalysisTool.aspx.

———. 2017b. "TCAB Framework." http://www.ihi.org/Engage/Initiatives/Completed/TCAB/Pages/Framework.aspx.

———. 2017c. "Transforming Care at the Bedside: Overview." http://www.ihi.org/engage/initiatives/completed/TCAB/Pages/default.aspx.

Institute of Medicine. 1983. *Nursing and Nursing Education: Public Policy and Private Actions.* Washington, DC: National Academies Press.

———. 2001. *Crossing the Quality Chasm: A New Health System for the 21st Century.* Washington, DC: National Academies Press.

———. 2003. *The Future of the Public's Health in the 21st Century.* Washington, DC: National Academies Press.

———. 2005. *Quality through Collaboration: The Future of Rural Health.* Washington, DC: National Academies Press.

———. 2006a. *Emergency Medical Services at the Crossroads.* Washington, DC: National Academies Press.

———. 2006b. *Improving the Quality of Healthcare for Mental and Substance-Use Conditions.* Washington, DC: National Academies Press.

———. 2007a. *Emergency Care for Children: Growing Pains.* Washington, DC: National Academies Press.

———. 2007b. *Future of Emergency Care in the United States Health System.* Washington, DC: National Academies Press.

———. 2007c. *Hospital-Based Emergency Care: At the Breaking Point.* Washington, DC: National Academies Press.

———. 2008. *Retooling for an Aging America: Building the Healthcare Workforce.* Washington, DC: National Academies Press.

———. 2010a. *Redesigning Continuing Education in the Health Professions.* Washington, DC: National Academies Press.

———. 2010b. *A Summary of the February 2010 Forum on the Future of Nursing: Education.* Washington, DC: National Academies Press.

———. 2011a. *The Future of Nursing: Leading Change, Advancing Health.* Washington, DC: National Academies Press.

———. 2011b. *Health IT and Patient Safety: Building Safer Systems for Better Care.* Washington, DC: National Academies Press.

———. 2011c. *Leading Health Indicators for Healthy People 2020: Letter Report.* Washington, DC: National Academies Press.

———. 2011d. *Relieving Pain in America: A Blueprint for Transforming Prevention, Care, Education, and Research.* Washington, DC: National Academies Press.

———. 2014. *Dying in America: Improving Quality and Honoring Individual Preferences Near the End of Life.* Washington, DC: National Academies Press.

Institute for Safe Medication Practices. 2007. "Error-Prone Conditions that Lead to Student Nurse-Related Errors." ISMP Medication Safety Alert! Acute Care newsletter, October 18. https://www.ismp.org/newsletters/acutecare/articles/20071018.asp.

Interprofessional Education Collaborative Expert Panel. 2011. *Core Competencies for Interprofessional Collaborative Practice.* Washington, DC: Interprofessional Education Collaborative. www.aacn.nche.edu/education-resources/IPECReport.pdf.

iSixSigma. 2017a. "Benchmarking." Dictionary. https://www.isixsigma.com/dictionary/benchmarking/

———. 2017b. "Six Sigma." Dictionary. https://www.isixsigma.com/dictionary/six-sigma/.

Issenberg, S., W. McGaghie, E. Petrusa, D. Gordon, and R. Scalese. 2005. "Features and Uses of High-Fidelity Medical Simulations that Lead to Effective Learning: A BEME Systematic Review." *Medical Teacher* 27:10–28.

The Joint Commission. 2007. *"What Did the Doctor Say?": Improving Health Literacy to Protect Patient Safety.* Health Care at the Crossroads series. Oakbrook Terrace, IL: The Joint Commission. http://www.jointcommission.org/What_Did_the_Doctor_Say.

———. 2011. "Healthcare Worker Fatigue and Patient Safety." *The Joint Commission Sentinel Event Alert* 48:1–3.

———. 2016. "Speak Up Initiatives." https://www.jointcommission.org/speakup.aspx.

Jones, D., M. DeVita, and R. Bellomo. 2011. "Rapid-Response Teams." *New England Journal of Medicine* 365:139–46.

Kahn, M. 2008. "Etiquette-Based Medicine." *New England Journal of Medicine* 358 (19): 1988–89.

Kalisch, B. 2015. *Errors of Omission: How Missed Nursing Care Imperils Patients.* Silver Spring, MD: American Nurses Association.

Kalisch, B., S. Begeny, and C. Anderson. 2008. "The Effect of Consistent Nursing Shifts on Teamwork and Continuity of Care." *Journal of Nursing Administration* 38 (3): 132–37.

Kaplan, G., M. Hamilton Lopez, and J. M. McGinnis, eds. 2015. *Transforming Health Care Scheduling and Access: Getting to Now.* Washington, DC: National Academies Press.

Ketchum, K., C. Grass, and A. Padwojski. 2005. "Medication Reconciliation." *American Journal of Nursing* 105 (11): 78–85.

Kohn, L., J. Corrigan, and M. Donaldson, eds. 1999. *To Err Is Human: Building a Safer Health System.* Washington, DC: National Academies Press.

Koplan, J., C. Liverman, and V. Kraak, eds. 2005. *Preventing Childhood Obesity: Health in the Balance.* Washington, DC: National Academies Press.

Kovner, A., and T. Rundall. 2009. "Evidence-Based Management Reconsidered." In *Evidence-Based Management in Health Care,* edited by A. Kovner, D. Fine, and R. D'Aquila, 53–77. Chicago: Health Administration Press.

Kronick, R. 2015. "New AHRQ Report Shows Patient Safety and Access Improvements, but Disparities Remain." *AHRQ Views* (blog), April. http://www.ahrq.gov/news/blog/ahrqviews/042015.html

Kurtzman, E., and P. Buerhaus. 2008. "New Medicare Payment Rules: Danger or Opportunity for Nursing." *American Journal of Nursing* 108 (6): 30–35.

Kutney-Lee, A., and K. Deena. 2011. "The Effect of Hospital Electronic Health Record Adoption on Nurse-Assessed Quality of Care and Patient Safety." *Journal of Nursing Administration* 41 (11): 466–72.

Leape, L. L. 1994. "Error in Medicine." *Journal of the American Medical Association* 272 (23): 1851–57. http://www.uphs.upenn.edu/gme/pdfs/Leape_Error%20in%20 Medicine_JAMA.pdf.

Leape, L. L., T. Brennan, N. Laird, A. G. Lawthers, R. Localio, B. A. Barnes, L. Hebert et al. 1991. "The Nature of Adverse Events in Hospitalized Patients—Results of the Harvard Medical Practice Study II." *New England Journal of Medicine* 324:377–84.

Lewis, N. 2011. "EHR Adoption to Reach 80% by 2016." *InformationWeek Healthcare*, November 28. http://informationweek.com/news/healthcare/EMR/232200275.

Lohr, K., ed. 1990. *Medicare: A Strategy for Quality Assurance.* 2 vols. Washington, DC: National Academies Press.

Long, K. 2003. "The Institute of Medicine Report: *Health Professions Education: A Bridge to Quality." Policy, Politics, & Nursing Practice* 4 (4): 259–62.

Maeshiro, R., C. Evans, J. Stanley, S. Meyer, V. Spolsky, S. Shannon, M. Bigley, J. Allan, W. Lang, and K. Johnson. 2011. "Using the Clinical Prevention and Population Health Curriculum Framework to Encourage Curricular Change." *American Journal of Preventive Medicine* 40 (2): 232–44.

Manno, M. 2006. "Preventing Adverse Drug Events." *Nursing* 36 (3): 56–61.

Manojlovich, M., and A. Talsma. 2007. "Identifying Nursing Processes to Reduce Failure to Rescue." *Journal of Nursing Administration* 37 (11): 504–9.

Marrelli, T. 2016. *Home Care Nursing: Surviving in an Ever-Changing Care Environment.* Indianapolis: Sigma Theta Tau International.

Marshall, D. 2008. "Evidence-Based Management." *Journal of Nursing Administration* 38 (5): 205–7.

Martin, S., P. Greenhouse, T. Merryman, J. Shovel, C. Liberi, and J. Konzier. 2007. "Transforming Care at the Bedside: Implementation and Spread Model for Single-Hospital and Multihospital Systems." *Journal of Nursing Administration* 37 (10): 444–51.

Mason, D. 2004. "Who Says It's an Error?" *American Journal of Nursing* 104 (6): 7.

McCloskey, J., and G. Bulechek, eds. 2000. *Nursing Interventions Classification.* St. Louis: Mosby.

McCoy, M., and V. Weisfeld, eds. 2015. *Future Directions of Credentialing Research in Nursing: Workshop Summary.* Washington, DC: National Academies Press.

Medicare.gov. 2016. "30-Day Unplanned Readmission and Death Measures." https:// www.medicare.gov/hospitalcompare/Data/30-day-measures.html.

Minority Nurse Staff. 2013. "Using Evidence-Based Practice to Improve Minority Health Outcomes." *Minority Nurse*, March 30. http://minoritynurse.com/ using-evidence-based-practice-to-improve-minority-health-outcomes/.

Montalvo, I., and N. Dunton. 2007. *Transforming Nursing Data into Quality Care: Profiles of Quality Improvement in U.S. Healthcare Facilities.* Silver Spring, MD: American Nurses Association.

Morjikian, R., and J. Bellack. 2005. "The RWJ Executive Nurses Fellows Program, Part 1." *Journal of Nursing Administration* 35 (10): 431–38.

Morton, P. 1995. "Creating a Laboratory that Simulates the Critical Care Environment." *Critical Care Nurse* 16 (16): 76–81.

Mozes, A. 2008. "Health Insurance Premiums Skyrocket." *HealthDay News*, April 29. http://i.abcnews.com/Health/Healthday/Story?id=4747936&page=3

National Center for Complementary and Integrative Health. 2015. "Americans Are in Pain: Analysis of Data on the Prevalence and Severity of Pain from National Survey." National Institutes of Health, August 11. https://nccih.nih.gov/research/results/spotlight/081515.

National Center for Medical Home Implementation. 2017. "What Is Medical Home?" https://medicalhomeinfo.aap.org/overview/Pages/Whatisthemedicalhome.aspx.

National Coordinating Council for Medication Error Reporting and Prevention. 2008. "Statement on Medication Error Rates." http://www.nccmerp.org/statement-medication-error-rates.

National Council of State Boards of Nursing. 2005. *Clinical Instruction in Prelicensure Nursing Programs.* NCSBN Position Paper. Chicago: National Council of State Boards of Nursing.

———. 2013. "Meeting the Ongoing Challenge of Continued Competence." https://www.ncsbn.org/Continued_Comp_Paper_TestingServices.pdf.

———. 2015. "Transition to Practice: Study Results." https://www.ncsbn.org/6889.htm.

———. 2016a. "Delegation." https://www.ncsbn.org/1625.htm.

———. 2016b. "Practice Error and Risk Factors (TERCAP)." https://www.ncsbn.org/113.htm.

National Institute of Nursing Research. 2016. *Advancing Science, Improving Lives: A Vision for Nursing Science.* Bethesda, MD: National Institutes of Health. https://www.ninr.nih.gov/sites/www.ninr.nih.gov/files/NINR_StratPlan2016_reduced.pdf.

National Institutes of Health. 2014. "Interdisciplinary Research." http://commonfund.nih.gov/interdisciplinary/overview.aspx.

———. 2014. "HHS Leaders Call for Expanded Use of Medications to Combat Opioid Overdose Epidemic." News release, April 24. https://www.nih.gov/news-events/news-releases/hhs-leaders-call-expanded-use-medications-combat-opioid-overdose-epidemic.

Naylor, M., A. Lustig, H. Kelley, E. Volpe, L. Melichar, and M. Pauly. 2013. "Introduction: The Interdisciplinary Nursing Quality Research Initiative." *Medical Care* 51 (4): S1–S5.

Nehring, W., W. Ellis, and F. Lashely. 2001. "Human Patient Simulators in Nursing Education: An Overview." *Simulation & Gaming* 32: 194–204.

Newhouse, R. 2008. "Evidence-Based Behavioral Practice: An Exemplar of Interprofessional Collaboration." *Journal of Nursing Administration* 38 (10): 414–16.

Nielsen-Bohlman, L., A. Panzer, and D. Kindig, eds. 2004. *Health Literacy: A Prescription to End Confusion.* Washington, DC: National Academies Press.

Nurse.com. 2008. "'Just Culture' System for Nurses Takes Focus of Medical Errors from Penalties to Solutions." March 10. https://www.nurse.com/blog/2008/03/10/just-culture-system-for-nurses-takes-focus-of-medical-errors-from-penalties-to-solutions-2/.

Obama, B. 2016. "United States Healthcare Reform Progress to Date and Next Steps." *Journal of the American Medical Association* 316 (5): 525–32.

Office of the National Coordinator for Health Information Technology. 2015. *Federal Health IT Strategic Plan 2015-2020.* https://www.healthit.gov/sites/default/files/9-5-federalhealthitstratplanfinal_0.pdf.

Olson, S., ed. 2011. *Allied Health Workforce and Services: Workshop Summary.* Washington, DC: National Academies Press.

———, ed. 2016. *Obesity in the Early Childhood Years: State of the Science and Implementation of Promising Solutions: Workshop in Brief.* Washington, DC: National Academies Press.

Olson, L., C. Grossmann, and J. M. McGinnis, eds. 2011. *Learning What Works: Infrastructure Required for Comparative Effectiveness Research: Workshop Summary.* Washington, DC: National Academies Press.

Olson, S., and N. Keren, eds. 2015. *Opportunities to Promote Children's Behavioral Health: Health Care Reform and Beyond: Workshop Summary.* Washington, DC: National Academies Press.

O'Neil, E., and M. Chow. 2011. "Leadership Action for a New American Health System." *Nurse Leader* 9 (6): 34–37.

Orlando Business Journal. 2008. "250,000 More Healthcare Workers Needed By 2020." February 29. http://www.bizjournals.com/orlando/stories/2008/02/25/daily37.html.

Pappas, S. 2008. "The Cost of Nurse-Sensitive Adverse Events." *Journal of Nursing Administration* 38 (5): 230–36.

Patient Safety Network. 2015a. "Medication Errors." Patient Safety Primer, March. https://psnet.ahrq.gov/primers/primer/23/medication-errors.

———. 2015b. "Medication Reconciliation." Patient Safety Primer, March. https://psnet.ahrq.gov/primers/primer/1.

———. 2016a. "Adverse Events after Discharge." Patient Safety Primer, July. http://psnet.ahrq.gov/primer.aspx?primerID=11.

———. 2016b. "Wrong-Site, Wrong-Procedure, and Wrong-Patient Surgery." Patient Safety Primer, July. https://psnet.ahrq.gov/primers/primer/18/wrong-site-wrong-procedure-and-wrong-patient-surgery.

Pfeffer, J., and R. Sutton. 2006. "Evidence-Based Management." *Harvard Business Review* 84:62–74.

Pianin, E. 2015. "US Healthcare Costs Surge to 17 Percent of GNP." *Fiscal Times, December 3.* http://www.thefiscaltimes.com/2015/12/03/Federal-Health-Care-Costs-Surge-17-Percent-GDP.

Pollard, P., K. Mitra, and D. Mendelson. 1996. *Nursing Report Card for Acute Care.* Washington, DC: American Nurses Publishing.

Puchner, L. 1995. "Literacy Links: Issues in the Relationship between Early Childhood Development, Health, Women, Families, and Literacy." *International Journal of Educational Development* 15 (3): 307–19.

Pulley, J. 2008. "What Nurses Want." *HealthcareIT News,* March 13. http://www.healthcareitnews.com/news/what-nurses-want.

Politico Staff. 2009. "Obama-Care 101: The President's 8 Principles." *Politico,* February 26. http://www.politico.com/story/2009/02/obama-care-101-the-presidents-8-principles-019362.

Reason, J. 1990. *Human Error.* Cambridge, UK: Cambridge University Press.

Resar, R., and L. Midelfort. 2008. "Medication Reconciliation Review." Institute for Health Improvement. http://www.ihi.org/knowledge/Pages/Tools/MedicationReconciliationReview.aspx.

Rivara, P., and S. Le Menestrel, eds. 2016. *Preventing Bullying through Science, Policy and Practice.* Washington, DC: National Academies Press.

Robert, N., and S. Finlayson. 2015. *Fundamentals of Magnet Toolkit.* Silver Spring, MD: American Nurses Association.

Robert Wood Johnson Foundation. 2007. *A Summary of the Impact of Reforms to the Hospital Inpatient Prospective Payment System (IPPS) on Nursing Services.* https://www3.centrahealth.com/pdf/LilleehandoutI.pdf.

———. 2008. "Demands on Nurses Grow as Hospital Quality Improvement Activities Increase." March 20. http://www.rwjf.org/en/library/articles-and-news/2008/03/demands-on-nurses-grow-as-hospital-quality-improvement-activitie.html.

Rogers, A., W.-T. Hwang, L. Scott, L. Aiken, and D. Dinges. 2004. "The Working Hours of Hospital Staff Nurses and Patient Safety." *Health Affairs* 23 (4): 202–12.

Rudd, R. 2013. Public Health Literacy. PowerPoint presented at the Institute of Medicine Workshop on Implication of Health Literacy for Public Health, Irvine, California, November 21. https://www.ncbi.nlm.nih.gov/books/NBK242431/.

Rural Health Information Hub. 2016. "Rural Health Disparities." https://www.ruralhealthinfo.org/topics/rural-health-disparities.

Sackett, D., W. Rosenberg, and M. Gray. 1996. "Evidence Based Medicine: What It Is and What It Isn't." *British Medical Journal* 312:71–72.

Salisbury, J., and S. Byrd. 2006. "Why Diversity Matters in Healthcare." *California Society of Anesthesiologists Bulletin*, Spring. http://www.csahq.org/pdf/bulletin/issue_12/Diversity.pdf.

Salmon, M. 2007. "Guest Editorial: Care Quality and Safety: Same Old?" *Nursing Outlook* 55 (3): 117–19.

Schaeffer, L., A. Schultz, and J. Salerno, eds. 2009. *HHS in the 21st Century: Charting a New Course for a Healthier America*. Washington, DC: The National Academies Press.

Seyda, B., T. Shelton, and N. DiVenere. 2008. "Family-Centered Care: Why It Is Important, How to Provide It, and What Parents And Children Are Doing to Make It Happen." In Earp, French, and Gilkey, *Patient Advocacy*, 61–91.

Shalala, D., and B. Vladeck. 2011. "Leading Change: How Nurses can Attract Political Support for the IOM Report on the Future of Nursing." *Nurse Leader* 9 (6): 38–39, 45.

Shea, K., A. Shih, and K. Davis. 2007. *Health Care Opinion Leaders' Views on the Quality and Safety of Health Care in the United States*. New York: Commonwealth Fund.

Sigma Theta Tau International, eds. 2006. *Resources for Implementing Evidence-Based Nursing*. Nurse Advance Collection. Indianapolis: Author.

Simmons, B. 2010. "Clinical Reasoning: Concept Analysis." *Journal of Advanced Nursing* 66:1151–58.

Siserhen, L., R. Blaszak, M. Woods, and C. Smith. 2007. "Defining Family-Centered Rounds." *Teaching and Learning in Medicine* 19 (3): 319–22.

Sitterding, M. 2015. "An Overview of Information Overload." In Sitterding and Broome, *Information Overload*, 1–9.

Sitterding, M., and M. Broome, eds. 2015. *Information Overload: Framework, Tips, and Tools to Manage in Complex Healthcare Environments*. Silver Spring, MD: American Nurses Association.

Sitterding, M., and P. Ebright. 2015. "Information Overload: A Framework for Explaining the Issues and Creating Solutions." In Sitterding and Broome, *Information Overload*, 11–33.

Slavitt, A. 2016. Comments at the J.P. Morgan 34th Annual Health Care Conference, San Francisco, California, January 11–15. http://medtecheng.com/comments-of-cms-acting-administrator-andy-slavitt-at-the-j-p-morgan-annual-health-care-conference-jan-11-2016/

Smedley, B., A. Stith, and A. Nelson, eds. 2003. *Unequal Treatment: Confronting Racial and Ethnic Disparities in Health Care*. Washington, DC: National Academies Press.

Smith, J., and L. Crawford. 2003. *Report of Findings from the Practice and Professional Issues Survey*. NCSBN Research Brief vol. 7. Chicago: National Council of State Boards of Nursing.

Spath, P. 2008. "Safety from the Patient's Point of View." In *Engaging Patients as Safety Partners*, edited by P. Spath, 1–34. Chicago: AHA Press.

Speakman, E., in collaboration with E. Tagliareni, A. Sherburne, and S. Sicks. 2015. *Guide to Effective Interprofessional Education Experiences in Nursing Education*. http://www.nln.org/docs/default-source/default-document-library/ipe-toolkit-krk-012716.pdf?sfvrsn=6.

Spear, S. 2005. "Fixing Healthcare from the Inside, Today." *Harvard Business Review*, September, 78–91.

Sullivan, L. 2004. *Missing Persons: Minorities in the Health Professions*. N.p.: The Sullivan Commission. http://health-quity.pitt.edu/40/1/Sullivan_Final_Report_000.pdf.

Swanson, K., and D. Wojnar. 2004. "Optimal Healing Environments in Nursing." *Journal of Alternative and Complementary Medicine* 10 (1): S-43–S-48.

Swift, E., ed. 2002. *Guidance for the National Healthcare Disparities Report*. Washington, DC: National Academies Press.

Tanner, C. 2003. "Building the Bridge to Quality." *Journal of Nursing Education* 42 (1): 431–32.

Trossman, S. 2011. "The Practice of Ethics." *American Nurse Today* 6 (11): 32–33.

Vincent, C., and A. Coulter. 2002. "Patient Safety: What about the Patient?" *Quality and Safety in Healthcare* 11:76–80.

Wagner, E. 1998. "Chronic Disease Management: What Will It Take to Improve Care for Chronic Illness?" *Effective Clinical Practice* 1:2–4.

Wakefield, M. 1997. "Pioneering New Ways to Ensure Quality Healthcare." *Nursing Economics* 15 (4): 225–27.

Weick , K. 2009. *Making Sense of the Organization. New York: John Wiley & Sons.*

Weisfeld, V., and T. Lustig, eds. 2015. *The Future of Home Health Care: Workshop Summary*. Washington, DC: National Academies Press.

White House. 2016. "Fact Sheet: Obama Administration Announces Additional Actions to Address the Prescription Opioid Abuse and Heroin Epidemic." March 29. https://obamawhitehouse.archives.gov/the-press-office/2016/03/29/fact-sheet-obama-administration-announces-additional-actions-address.

White, K., and A. O'Sullivan, eds. 2012. *The Essential Guide to Nursing Practice. Applying ANA's Scope and Standards in Practice and Education.* Silver Spring, MD: American Nurses Association.

Wilson-Stronks, A., K. Lee, C. Cordero, A. Kopp, and E. Galvez. 2008. *One Size Does Not Fit All: Meeting the Healthcare Needs of Diverse Populations*. Oakbrook Terrace, IL: The Joint Commission. http://www.jointcommission.org/assets/1/6/HLCOneSizeFinal.pdf.

Wilson-Stronks, A., P. Schyve, C. Cordero, I. Rodriguez, and M. Youdelman. 2010. *Advancing Effective Communication, Cultural Competence, and Patient- and Family-Centered Care: A Roadmap for Hospitals*. Oakbrook Terrace, IL: The Joint Commission. https://www.jointcommission.org/assets/1/6/ARoadmapforHospitalsfinalversion727.pdf.

Wizemann, T., and D. Thompson, eds. 2015a. *The Role and Potential of Communities in Population Health Improvement: Workshop Summary*. Washington, DC: National Academies Press.

———, eds. 2015b. *Spread, Scale, and Sustainability in Population Health: Workshop Summary*. Washington, DC: National Academies Press.

Wolf, Z. 2001. "Understanding Medication Errors." *Nursing Spectrum Metro Edition*, May, 31–33.

World Health Organization. 2010. *Framework for Action on Interprofessional Education and Collaborative Practice*. Geneva: World Health Organization. http://www.who.int/hrh/resources/framework_action/en/index.html.

———. 2016a. "Social Determinants of Health." http://www.who.int/social_determinants/en/

———. 2016b. *World Health Statistics 2016: Monitoring Health for the SDGs. Geneva: WHO Press*. http://www.who.int/gho/publications/world_health_statistics/2016/en/

World Health Organization. 2008. "Adverse Events." WHO Collaborating Centre for Patient Safety Solutions. http://www.who.int/patientsafety/solutions/patientsafety/collaborating_centre/en/.

Index